What readers and medical professionals are saying...

"In a single book, Dr. Sasse has given all of us a proven blueprint for succeeding at losing weight and transforming our lives. Funny, practical, and backed by impeccable science, *Life-Changing Weight Loss* delivers the goods. I defy anyone to pick up this book and not find it absolutely fascinating and inspiring."

—*Robert Watson, MD, Fellow of the American College of Surgeons*

"Inspiring and thought provoking, *Life-Changing Weight Loss* not only gives us the inspiration to succeed at losing weight, but it also provides the proven and clear step-by-step approach on how to do it. Finally, a weight-loss guide that actually guides us to lose weight."

—*Brie Moore, PhD, Clinical Psychologist*

"After you read *Life-Changing Weight Loss*, your life will never be the same. You will approach your diet, your health, and your life in a completely new and more positive way. This book gives you all the tools you need to succeed at losing weight and changing your life for the better."

—*Gayl Fording, RN*

Life-Changing Weight Loss

Feel More Energetic and Live a More Active Life
with a Proven, Medically Based
Weight Loss Program

A SASSE GUIDE™

Kent Sasse, MD, MPH, FACS

360 PUBLISHING

Reno, Nevada

360° Publishing, LLC.
3495 Lakeside Drive, Suite 205
Reno, NV 89509
www.sasseguide.com

Book Cover and Page Layout: Anita Jones, Another Jones Graphics

Visit Dr. Sasse's Web site at www.sasseguide.com

Publisher's Cataloging-In-Publication Data
(Prepared by The Donohue Group, Inc.)

Sasse, Kent.
   Life-changing weight loss : feel more energetic and live a more active life with a proven, medically based weight loss program / Kent Sasse.

   p. ; cm. -- (Sasse guide)

   Includes bibliographical references and index.
   ISBN: 978-1-934727-23-2

1. Weight loss--Popular works. 2. Weight loss--Psychological aspects--Popular works. 3. Reducing diets--Popular works. 4. Reducing exercises--Popular works. I. Title.

RM222.2 .S271 2010
613.2/5

Printed in the United States

CONTENTS

DEDICATION

To Henry Sasse, who taught me to be unafraid and from whom I learned to work hard for change.

ACKNOWLEDGMENTS

I AM DEEPLY indebted to so many people who have helped to make this book possible and who have helped in its research and writing. First and foremost, I would like to thank my patients, who perform the daily miracles of fighting this disease of obesity and who challenge me and my colleagues to be better caregivers and better people.

I am indebted to so many people at the International Metabolic Institute and Western Bariatric Institute for their hard work and dedication to our patients and to the work of combating this disease. To Sarai Swanson, Roberta Brown, Kimberly Brown, Donna Wainscoat, Jennifer Padgett, Trees Lonis-Muller, Patrick Allen, Gayleen Gott-Anderson, Curtis Smith, Darolyn Skelton, Laramie Lathrop, Laurie McGinley, Marte Lyson, Mason Hermosillo, Nicole Walker, Vicki Bovee, Dr. Kozar, Dr. Ganser, Dr. Watson, Cindi Lee, Gregory Bowman, Mark Conte, Tracy Visher, Natasha Mulqueen, Dr. Pamela Corson, Doina Kulick, Dr. Michael Bloch, Dr. Kristina Hansen, Stephen Mayville, PhD, Brie Moore, PhD, Dennis Fitzpatrick, Robin Marquez, RN, Erin Wallace, and Corey Moore.

Jennifer Baumer, Cindie Geddes, Jessie Gardner and Anita Jones have done an amazing job of editing and designing this book. Dionne Lim has been an outstanding research assistant and investigator of facts. I would also like to thank Craig Belis, Jason Green, Joanne McCall, and Sharon Castlen for their hard work, patience, dedication, and sense of humor.

FOREWORD

Around the world today, more people than ever wish to change their lives. More importantly, more people than ever need to change their lives by losing weight. Increasingly, individuals find that they are not able to live the lives they have imagined and live up to their potential because of weight gain that has sapped their energy, limited their opportunities, and diminished their quality of life. For decades, physicians, dietitians, and psychologists have struggled with the development of effective tools to produce and maintain weight loss. Dr. Sasse's *Life-Changing Weight Loss* is one such resource that is focused so precisely and so compellingly on the true method by which a person can successfully achieve lasting weight loss: through personal life change.

Dr. Sasse is one of the nation's thought leaders in medically based weight loss who offers a compelling and real-world practical guide for losing weight and transforming your life. It is the perfect synthesis of empirically based research findings and real-world applied experience that makes Dr. Sasse's *Life-Changing Weight Loss* the essential weight-loss resource.

Have you wanted to lose weight? Have you tried diets and exercise programs and commercial centers, only to find that you have regained the pounds later? If so, understand that you hold in your hands a solution that can help you bring about positive life change. And, as is demonstrated by the testimonials from real-life patients who have sought out Dr. Sasse's medical weight loss center, the method is derived from experience. Dr. Sasse offers a practical and well-reasoned approach to dietary modification that still allows for enjoyable eating and living while emphasizing effective ways to cut calories and reduce body fat. He focuses on research-proven nutritional science, not on fad diets or gimmicks that might help you to lose weight for a brief period of time. So many of us have become tired of the promises from flash-in-the-pan diet programs that produce some short-term weight loss. Here is the "real deal" for long-term sustained weight loss.

As Dr. Sasse emphasizes, in order to make the change permanent and to really transform your life into a healthier one that offers you greater quality of life and increased energy, you must not only change your diet, but you must also change your life. This journey of personal life change embraces a change in knowledge, attitude, and all of the other factors of diet, eating behaviors, and exercise.

Dr. Sasse walks you through the elements of life change, including the need to accept responsibility for the change, the importance of committing to short-term goals and long-term goals, and the benefits of breaking down the project into many small, achievable steps. He not only tells you what is necessary to make this vitally important life change, but he also gives you the tools you need to do so successfully and effectively.

Life Changing Weight Loss is truly a unique, breakthrough book in the science of weight loss. And it could not have come at a better and more critically important time, when so many people are in need of a proven method for sustained weight loss. Without losing pounds, few of us can live up to our potential.

With this book and the methods that are outlined in it, you can make the change and succeed for a lifetime.

Stephen B. Mayville, PhD, BCBA
Licensed Clinical Psychologist
Director of Psychological Services
International Metabolic Institute

INTRODUCTION

Congratulations! If you picked up this book because you've made a commitment to making permanent changes in your life by losing weight and becoming healthier, good for you! You've already taken the first step on the road to change. If you picked up this book because someone you love is overweight and you want to help in the battle against excessive weight and the health complications it causes, then you will find this book an invaluable resource.

I am committed to helping people who need to lose weight. As a physician and surgeon specializing in weight loss, I have helped thousands of people succeed at losing weight through medically based weight-loss programs and weight-loss surgery. As founder of the International Metabolic Institute™ (iMetabolic®) and Western Bariatric Institute in Reno, Nevada, I've had the great privilege of successfully guiding thousands of people to lose weight and keep it off. I've learned from their experiences what works, and what doesn't, in weight loss.

My commitment comes from having listened to the life stories of the amazing people I see in my practice every day. By listening carefully to their personal stories and fighting alongside my patients in this battle, I've gained a deep understanding of what it's like to struggle against insidious weight gain, and what it's like to conquer it. I've come to understand how hard it is for anyone to lose weight and to keep it off and how great it feels to achieve those goals. I know the statistics; I understand how steeply the odds are stacked against anyone who embarks on this journey all alone, without help.

From the beginning of my practice, I've had patients tell me they'd lost and gained the same 25 pounds over and over. Then, as my practice grew, I began to see it for myself. The diets, systems, and drugs they were using worked for a short period but not over time. I knew there had to be a better way—a way to make weight loss permanent.

Today the vast majority of people who struggle with weight gain do so in a society packed with opportunities and pressures to overeat high-calorie, high-carbohydrate food. Today's world is fast paced with plenty of fast food, and those people who make time to work out are applauded—right up until it's time to schedule a meeting that conflicts with that workout. As soon as your commitment conflicts with what someone else might want from you, that applause goes out the window.

By researching weight loss and studying the most successful techniques from the most successful weight-loss centers in the world, I began to see solutions for that repetitive weight gain–weight loss cycle.

What I learned both challenged and inspired me because I soon learned that solutions weren't easy to come by. I learned from the best and most successful programs, observed the immense value of a medically based approach, and saw that conscious life change that incorporates nutrition, exercise, and a structured program is the key to long-term weight-loss success. Real success must overcome years of obstacles both from within and from without. I became inspired to create the best, most effective, and most powerful weight-loss program in the world and bring it forward to help people change their lives.

This book is about the science of weight loss and personal change. It's not about hype. This book doesn't offer fad diets; it's about what works for real people in the real world. This book brings you a proven weight-loss program developed from science and medicine—that has been shaped and improved by the experiences of thousands before you.

The only way to lose the weight and keep it off is to change your life in the ways I describe in the chapters ahead. You *can* succeed at losing this weight and keeping it off for good. You *can* change your life as well as your weight. You *can* have the life you deserve.

This book will show you how.

Introduction

The Glamour of Getting Started

The popular diets—the ones that show up in glossy magazines and on talk shows; the ones dressed up with pretty pictures and familiar faces—often center around a single element, such as a single food group, vitamin, mineral, or vegetable. And they speak very little to the key elements of true-life change. Many catchy programs and fad diets capture the imagination of the public at large, while more sound solutions with medical backing—those that have been proven by years of scientific research, stud, and trials—lack the glamour and never catch the public's eye. Maybe it's because the medically proven, scientifically studied solutions often involve a variety of components that need to be combined in the right way in order to achieve success. Remembering that all you're having for breakfast, lunch, *and* dinner is carrots is easier than figuring out your calories and the food groups that account for them.

The trendy summer diets catch the eye. They seem glamorous; they're surrounded by hype and often endorsed by movie stars.

But they don't produce lasting change.

Only you can make the changes in your life that will stand the test of time. And you *can* do so—by reading this book carefully and following the principles it sets forth.

Through my role, as a medical director and bariatric surgeon, of helping people lose weight over the years, I've learned that the *real* glamour is in *success*—even if, or maybe *especially* if, the success is earned through hard work and commitment.

I have dedicated myself to researching, investigating, and reporting on effective, evidence-based weight-loss solutions and strategies. As I've watched my patients learn and succeed, I've found that their experiences match what I'm reading in the research—that no single, narrowly defined solution, diet, or technique is going to work for every single individual. The best weight-loss solutions are customized for individuals. The best solutions draw on evidence from all the disciplines that come into play with weight loss: behavioral medicine, psychology, fitness training, nutrition, bariatric surgery, and medical endocrinology. Evidence shows that programs that include information and techniques from each of these disciplines are more likely to help people find success than programs with more narrow parameters.

True success at losing weight and keeping it off means true success in changing your life for the better. Changing your life requires tapping into the deep desire for change you know you have in your soul. You must uncover the most powerful motivations that drive you to seek change: the desire for improved feelings of self-worth, heightened ability to perform physical activities, improved relationships, a better sex life, greater happiness in life, and better financial and professional opportunities. And you must draw strength from the power of those motivations as you begin your journey to a stronger, healthier, more satisfied new you.

YOUR WEIGHT-LOSS BOOK

This book is filled with medical science, tips, and advice that I've learned and gathered in my practice as a weight-loss physician. Together, that science, those tips, and the advice form the basis of the highly successful weight-loss program of this book. But your own experience is just as important. Throughout the book, I will be asking you questions about your life and your ideas. Get yourself a notebook or journal—one just for this project—and start recording your thoughts, opinions, feelings, and, yes, your answers to questions. This will become your weight-loss book, *your* road map to successful change. And it will be more important than anything I could write for you.

1

. . .

Choose to Change

Being even mildly overweight can produce discomfort, decreased energy, embarrassment, and low self-esteem for many people. Being more severely overweight can affect every aspect of one's life. According to studies, being overweight can even result in lower pay and fewer promotions at work. This is hardly fair, but it's too often true in a society that glamorizes lean figures.

Being seriously overweight plays havoc with a body. We simply aren't designed to be carrying around a bunch of extra weight. Our organs, our joints, our bones, even our brains–all eventually collapse under that weight. Given the health consequences that come from extra weight, losing that weight is a matter of life and death, especially for those seriously overweight people who have BMIs of more than 30. Being aware of the health consequences of being seriously overweight means living daily with the fear of potential medical complications. But being unaware of the consequences often means letting serious medical problems get out of hand. Ignorance is not bliss.

Just about everything is more difficult with extra weight, from walking up and down stairs to shopping for clothes. There's the daily physical toll of an aching back and joints. The lungs and heart must work harder than they are meant to. Plus there's the emotional toll that comes with the stigma of being overweight and enduring the comments made by people who don't understand but who take the opportunity to judge.

But what if you never had to worry about being overweight again?

Take a moment and consider what your life would be like if you weren't overweight. Imagine where you want to be, not just in three months, but also in six months; two years; ten years; twenty. Imagine the things you want to be doing and the people with whom you want to spend time. Think of all those things and put those into your heart now. Make them a part of your mind and your life. What kind of clothes would you buy? How would you change your life? How would you feel about yourself? What new job might you ponder applying for? Are there activities you've stopped participating in or never participated in that you'd like to try? Places you'd like to visit that you've never visited because it just seemed physically too hard to get there? Imagine if your weight no longer stopped you from pursuing your dreams. Wouldn't that make working for those dreams worthwhile?

What lies before us and what lies behind us are tiny matters compared to what lies within us.

— Oliver Wendell Holmes

Losing weight is a great achievement in and of itself. Your body will thank you. But so will your mind. Making the necessary changes in your life needed for losing weight, and then actually seeing the results of those changes, opens doors in your mind and prepares the way for other changes—some subtle; some not.. Being overweight, searching for a way out of weight gain and loss cycles, can be a sort of obsession. Your brain becomes so focused on this one issue that other concerns are drowned out. Once weight is removed from your list of concerns, your mind will start searching for other ways you might improve. And, because such a big change has been accomplished, your mind will find new confidence and a willingness to take on new challenges—and your body will finally be ready to rise to those challenges as well.

Now is the best time to create a clear mental picture of the person that you can become—the person inside you that flourishes in all you do and is no longer overweight. Whether this means seeing yourself without those extra 20 pounds and feeling more energetic or imagining yourself without the extra 125 pounds, no longer feeling short of breath and aching, and now able to volunteer with a group that matters to you, take a trip you've wanted to take, or accomplish any other goal, now is the time to picture it.

Live out of your imagination, not your history.
~ Stephen Covey

Picture it clearly. Don't limit yourself to a quick vision of what this would look like. Imagine each part of your body and how it would *feel*. See yourself engaging in activities you've always wanted to do or used to do. Imagine the sensory details—how it feels, what the sounds and sights and smells are, whom you interact with, what your day is like, what your achievements are, and what your goals have become.

No matter how qualified or deserving we are, we will never reach a better life until we can imagine it for ourselves and allow ourselves to have it.
~ Richard Bach

A good friend of mine who struggled with obesity for many years explained to me his epiphany one day. He came back from a spring picnic with his family and found himself alone in his study. His family had gone off for a hike along a stream, something that he did not feel physically up to doing. As he reflected on the beauty of the spring sunshine and the blossoming flowers and sounds of springs he'd witnessed that day, my friend realized that he missed being able to join his family on their hike and that he even resented those who could fully enjoy the day. For some reason, at that moment he saw with new clarity something very important about his life: he, and he alone, controlled and would determine the rest of that life.

In that moment he realized that the corollary to this epiphany was also true: Nobody else was going to make the sort of profound difference in his life that he could make. No one else was going to come to his rescue and immediately give him the *willpower*, the insight, and the tools necessary to improve his life.

He thought what life could be like if he were never overweight again, and he imagined enjoying that wonderful hike outdoors with his family where he felt he should be. He imagined all the other activities he would never again miss because of being too tired and overweight. In his case, he quite clearly understood that being overweight was the main impediment to his living a healthier and richer life

As he thought of that hike, he also was able to imagine what it would be like to enjoy all facets of his life more. He could spend more time with those he loved, have more satisfying relationships with his wife and children, and feel better about himself both mentally and physically. So much of what he wanted hinged on his being able to drop the excess pounds and maintain a healthy weight.

From that day forward, he vowed to make his own health his number one priority. He vowed to work on his goal of long-term weight loss and weight maintenance every single day for the rest of his life. No one else could do it with the same degree of dedication he could, and the realization inspired him.

He's kept his promise. Every day since that springtime afternoon, my friend has devoted time to working on this goal of long-term weight loss and maintenance. Some days he devotes a lot of time to it and makes time for significant physical activity, such as playing a vigorous tennis match or taking a long bike ride. Other days he checks his pedometer to see how many steps he's walked that day and reminds himself to park far away from the office in order to get in more steps. But no matter what day it is and no matter how many things he has going on, he keeps focused on his goal. Why? Because it's important *to him*. It's important for his health, his relationships, and his longevity, and he knows it.

I've watched people lose weight and gain charisma they never even knew they could have. There's always that one person at a party who attracts a lot of attention. Few people battling a serious weight problem have the ability to feel self-confident and outgoing–to project the confidence, warmth, and positive feelings that define charisma. Yes, there are exceptions, but overall, when you're struggling with a weight problem or another medical or personal problem, it's harder to project the breezy, friendly, charismatic warmth that draws others.

The qualities of self-confidence, positive attitude, warmth, and genuine caring for and interest in others are intrinsically linked to living at a normal body weight. It's natural and normal that, when you find yourself overweight, you're going to worry about your own health, feel more self-conscious in crowds, and spend more time in inward contemplation than outward exploration. It's natural to focus on the serious problems your weight is causing. Who has time or energy to worry about charisma?

You might be thinking you don't care about charisma, were never interested in being the life of the party, and just want to get rid of your weight problem–to which I say, "Amen; let's focus on the topic at hand." But keep in mind that all of those important qualities are linked, and know, too, that if you can follow the steps that lead to smart choices, commitment, and long-term weight loss, then you can enjoy benefits that go far beyond the relief of moving down a few clothing sizes. You can enjoy a greater sense of self-worth and self-confidence, and you may find that you are beginning to project more warmth and confidence to others as you become a naturally more charismatic you.

*I know the price of success: dedication, hard work, and an
unremitting devotion to the things you want to see happen.*
~ Frank Lloyd Wright

I asked you to imagine what you'd do with *your* new life. Now imagine
what it would be like for those people who love you. Imagine what it's like
for family and friends of people with limited mobility; people who have to
limit the events and activities in which they can participate. There are children who wish their parents could be more active in their sports; spouses
who want to pursue outdoor activities with their other halves; grandkids
who want their grandparents to have the energy and fitness to go river
rafting or to go river rafting with them or join them on vigorous hikes. If
there are people like this in your life, their love for you is undiminished
whether you're heavy or trim, but their experiences in life and their social
interactions with you would be and can be enriched when you become the
person you can be—someone at a healthier weight who is happier, stronger,
and more eager to participate in all the wonderful activities of life.

And life *can* be wonderful—if you're willing to put in the work. Stud-
ies show a very important relationship between obesity and depression.
People suffering from depression are more likely to become overweight.
And excess weight is a strong precursor to the development of depression.
It's a chicken-and-egg question, but the answer isn't as important as just
getting the proverbial "fowl" out of your life.

A number of fascinating studies have shown that a high percentage of
people who lose significant amounts of weight find that their depression
lifts. Body weight and body image are closely linked, and weight strongly
impacts mental self-image, depression or contentment, and self-esteem.
People are more apt to gain weight when they're depressed and more apt
to feel happier and less depressed when they lose weight. Sure, this is intui-
tively obvious—and no great surprise—to people who have already gained

and lost weight and experienced the roller coaster of self-doubt and depression that alternates with the sense of accomplishment and confidence at having lost weight. But it's always nice when science comes to common-sense conclusions.

Imagine moving to a *permanently* healthy weight and the feelings of satisfaction, accomplishment, and contentment you'll feel.

Dreams are renewable no matter what our age.

~ Dale Turner

Being overweight is a serious matter. It's not just about how you look. Overweight and obesity are chronic, life-threatening diseases. Did you know:

- Excessive body fat results in serious health problems over time.

- Being overweight puts a person at risk of more than 30 major medical conditions.

- Excess weight has medical, psychological, social, physical, and economic costs.

- A healthy BMI (a measure of body mass, e.g., weight) is approximately 18 to 25. A BMI of 25 or more signals *overweight.* A BMI of 30 signals *obesity.*

- The risk of diabetes rises rapidly when BMI surpasses 25. (Appendix A)

Only one in eleven people who are 100 pounds
overweight lives to age 65.
~ *New England Journal of Medicine*

WHY WE ARE OVERWEIGHT

The dawn of the 21st century presents people in our country and culture with a curious contradiction. With all the conveniences of the modern, technological world, the human race still functions with the same genes of our caveman ancestors.

Right now in the United States, there's a record 3,800 calories available to most Americans every day (compared to the approximately 2,300 we're supposed to have). Don't worry—most people aren't eating all of those calories. The 3,800 is just the number of calories available to us, meaning food that's available in the house, the office, the convenience store and fast food restaurant, and all the other places excess calories lurk. Some of those calories are lost when food goes bad or diners leave food on plates. But that still leaves a record number of calories being consumed by most people most days. That's a lot of food. An extra 500 calories a day equals one pound per week of weight gain. Over a year, that adds up fast. (See Appendix F for information on the specific dangers of weight gain and obesity.)

If you compare what we eat today to what we ate 40 years ago, you'll see a skyrocketing consumption of carbohydrates: sweets, sugars, high-fructose corn sweetener, cereals, grains, potatoes, and snacks. Consumption of these foods in the United States alone is at an all-time high.

But, while carbs are the worst offenders, we are consuming more calories of every kind. Meat consumption is also at a record high, with an average consumption of 195 pounds of red meat, poultry, and fish per person per year. We're also eating nearly 30 pounds of cheese each year. As a dairy product, cheese is packed with protein, which is good, but it's also full of fat and is high in calories.

Consider this:

- Americans eat approximately 200 pounds of flour and cereal products every year. That's 45 pounds more per person than in the 1950s.

- While we eat more than the recommended number of servings of grains every day, most people are still falling short on eating the healthy whole grains–those 45 pounds of grains and flour products are largely refined grains.

- The consumption of sugars and other sweeteners is skyrocketing. In 2000 Americans consumed an average of 152 pounds of caloric sweeteners per person.

The USDA recommends no more than 40 grams of sugar in an average daily diet of 2,500 calories–the equivalent of 10 teaspoons of sugar or one 12-ounce soda. But most people are getting a lot more than that, and it's not always on purpose–sugar shows up in many unlikely places, from ketchup to pizza, lunchmeat to canned vegetables. Unlikely culprits for additional sugar in a diet include yogurt, salad dressings, hot dogs, soups, and boxed flavored rice mixes. It's hard to avoid, even when people try. But the main sources are obvious: sweets, desserts, white flour, chips, snacks, potatoes, pasta, bread, and rice.

The challenges we face in maintaining a healthy weight aren't just limited to plentiful sources of high-carb, high-sugar foods. Issues of time and convenience also play major roles in our struggle. Sometimes it's just not possible to find healthy food in a hurry. But it is possible to find food. A lot of food. Food is everywhere–it's fast, easily accessible, convenient, and, thanks to focus groups, test kitchens, and added salt, sugar, seasonings, flavorings, and fat, it tastes very good. And it's available in convenience stores and fast food places, in handy boxed and frozen meals in grocery stores, and even through food delivery services. It's all been made so easy. Too easy.

Food has been made easier to find and to consume because so much of life has gotten harder. Most people are working harder, with longer hours and faster deadlines, which makes it hard to find time to make healthy, home-cooked meals and harder still to figure out all the ins and outs of nutrition in order to balance what a healthy body needs and the tasty snack that body craves. When there's time to cook, many people are cooking healthier than in the past, but those meals can be few and far between.

Fast Food, Fast Choices

Welcome to the world of convenience foods. Whether we grab a packaged frozen dinner or something from a fast food place, today it's easier than ever to pick up a fast, prepared meal that tastes good and satisfies our hunger (and that is also very high in calories, which our bodies then store as fat). Fast food joints are open late or round the clock, and they're fast, cheap, and convenient. All you have to do is pull up, order, drive through, and eat. You don't even have to get out of the car.

Fast food has also become more economical over the years. It's now often cheaper to pick up a fast food meal than to assemble all the ingredients and make one from scratch. But, cheap as it seems, fast food comes with a steep price tag: a huge number of calories and a huge load of carbohydrates–and you burned somewhere around zero calories getting it.

Fast Food, Slow Genetics

We live in a fast-paced, fast food, high-tech society in bodies that haven't changed appreciably since the Stone Age. Our genes still expect our bodies to work for food–to go out and chase down small game or wild boars or perform some other sort of hunter-gatherer behavior that's going to burn excess calories before we even secure any additional calories to burn. It's unlikely that there were many overweight cavemen. But is it any wonder that people today are gaining weight when the extent of the quest for food is a quarter-mile drive and a hand stuck out of the car window?

Not only are we not burning calories, but those caveman genes are programmed to hang on to every calorie the body gets. Our bodies have been genetically programmed to store every single calorie possible in case there is no more for a long time. While this may have been useful for the caveman, it's hurting those of us who have no fear of running out of food.

Human bodies actually have a highly efficient process in place for converting food to energy. Digestion begins the minute food is eaten, as the body breaks it down with enzymes and extracts nutrients for growth and calories for energy and stores whatever's not used for later. One of the ways calories are stored is as glycogen in the liver. Glycogen makes an easily accessible energy store that can be called upon quickly when needed. It's the second wind we tap when working out hard.

For long-term survival, as opposed to those short-term workouts, or in case the crops fail or the hunting-gathering goes poorly, our genes are still programmed to store energy in the form of fat in fat cells (or adipocytes) distributed throughout the body. Men tend to store fat around the waist and internally in the abdomen, while women tend to store it beneath the skin around the hips and thighs. Regardless of where the extra stores are kept, most of us don't want them! Our crops aren't all going to fail, and we're not literally hunting down our next meals. We'd just as soon not store every calorie we eat "just in case."

The average active adult should take in somewhere around 2,500 calories a day to maintain body weight (meaning to neither gain nor lose). But look at the impact of one fast food meal:

	CALORIES	FAT (GRAMS)	% CALORIES FAT	CARBS (GRAMS)
ORIGINAL DOUBLE WHOPPER, CHEESE, NO MAYO	900	51	51	53
SMALL FRIES	340	17	45	44
LARGE MILKSHAKE	950	39	37	151

After eating this one meal–call it lunch–there are only 410 calories left of those 2,500 to take care of the other meals, which might have already been consumed, and that's if you're trying to maintain weight and not lose.

A few facts on fast food.

- Every day, one in four Americans goes to a fast food restaurant.
- We now spend more than $110 billion on fast food annually.
- McDonald's feeds more than 46 million people daily– more than the entire population of Spain.
- Most nutritionists recommend not eating fast food more than once a month.

Source: http://supersizeme.com/home.aspx?page=bythelb

1 • CHOOSE TO CHANGE

THE POWER TO CHANGE

You have within you the power to change. And, while no one can do it for you, the wonderful fact is that it *can* be done–by you. You possess the unique human ability to change your circumstances, change jobs, develop new abilities, foster new talents, rid yourself of unwanted habits, and develop healthy ones in their place. You have the ability to change how you live and thereby change your life.

Despite the forces arrayed against you–the fast food industry, stress, hunger, constraints on time and energy from work, kids, home, and other duties, and the constant bombardment of advertisements and opportunities for food–you have the power and the ability to lose weight and improve your life.

> *The greatest discovery of my generation is that a human being can alter his life by altering his attitudes of mind.*
> ~ William James

Have you ever known anyone who quit smoking? There's a change! I've watched members of my own family quit smoking, and I can tell you there's nothing easy about it. Between the addictive properties of cigarettes and the powerful triggers from time of day and stress, cigarettes can be a killer to quit. But they're also a killer to start with. Though smoking is pleasurable, a smoker who quits does so knowing the price for the pleasure of smoking is just too high.

The process of breaking old habits and replacing them with new ones is the same for the smoker who quits and for the couch potato who hates exercise but decides to train for a marathon. Change requires choice. And choice can change anything.

13

It is not the strongest of the species that survives nor the most intelligent, but the one most responsive to change.

~ Charles Darwin

RESPONSIBILITY

No fairy godmother, magic spell, or perfect program can make the changes for you. Instead of focusing outward, you need to look inside and acknowledge the amazing truth: You have the power to change within you. You can change yourself. In fact, no one else can do it for you. With the magic of that realization comes responsibility.

While change is up to you, that doesn't mean you have to go it alone. One of the mottos of the International Metabolic Institute, where I work, is: *you can change. We can help.* And *Help* sums up the role of an expert, medically based weight-loss program.

A good weight-loss program or weight-loss center provides doctors and staff who are trained to provide powerful tools to help patients win the weight-loss battle once and for all. They can provide counseling, support groups, and proven methods for successful weight loss. A great weight-loss center can provide up-to-date information and tools, tips on avoiding food triggers, meal plans, healthy meal-replacement shakes, snacks, and bars that taste good, calorie calculators, inspirational messages, inspirational and informative books, and hundreds of other things that help in the battle. But only *you* can change.

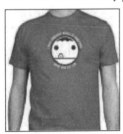

The antithesis of taking responsibility for your own change is the dark humor displayed on a T-shirt offered by the satirical humor magazine the *Onion*. The slogan on the shirt reads: "When is someone going to do something about how fat I am?"

On the face of it, the T-shirt is funny, but underneath? I've seen plenty of people who have realized there's a problem, but all too often they've blamed outside factors (an accident, an injury, a stressful job, a pregnancy, unexplained headaches or fatigue, to give just a few examples). They've come to understand they're hurting themselves with the extra weight, risking their health and hurting their families, but they still believe the solution must come from outside.

Sometimes the solution to problems does come from outside. I know very little about how my car works and I do approach it with a *please fix this* philosophy because I simply don't know how to fix a car myself. But it's still my responsibility to. But I still have the responsibility to know if the car is making strange noises or if the brakes seem to be wearing, and it's up to me to make the choice to take it to someone with the knowledge needed to get it back in working condition. Any mechanic will tell you that it helps if the customer has been paying attention, listening to the noises and noticing the way the car responds to braking. So, even though I don't understand how my car works, I'm not abdicating complete responsibility. When it comes to my health and managing my weight and fitness, I ask others for help and use their expertise, their experience, and the tools they provide. But I alone make the change.

The important thing is this: to be able at any moment to sacrifice what we are for what we could become.

~ Charles Dubois

Taking total responsibility for your weight-loss journey and the steps you're taking to get to your goals requires accepting that you're the only person who can get you to where you want to go. No one else understands how deeply important it is to you or what effects the extra weight have had on you as a person, and no one but you will experience as much reward when you reach your goals. Family and friends will cheer you on, and they'll be grateful when you take steps to improve your quality of life and your longevity, but ultimately they're not in your head. And they're not going to get the full impact of the joy, relief, and pride you'll feel as the weight comes off.

If you take responsibility for yourself, you will develop a hunger to accomplish your dreams.

~ Les Brown

Accepting total responsibility means looking in the mirror and acknowledging that where you are today is the result of your choices and actions in the past. Only by making changes in those choices and actions are you going to be able to look in the mirror in the future and see a different you—one in which you are proud.

Of course, this ownership of change also means ownership of any setbacks, failures, or lapses along the way. No one is force-feeding you. No one but you can decide there's no room for even 15 minutes of exercise in a busy day.

Total responsibility means taking responsibility for both the negatives and the positives—but, in the process, every setback needs to become a learning opportunity. What did you do wrong? What could you have done differently? Are you on a plateau? Do you understand how to jump-start your weight loss again? At the same time, every step forward is a milestone that deserves celebration and notice. What did you do right? Can you do it again? Where did the willpower come from?

Of course, thousands of external factors also contribute to your successes or failures, but it's your decision to let a busy day blow your workout or to turn a quick dinner into a caloric nightmare. You may have inherited lousy genes or degenerative joints or any of a vast array of hurdles to overcome, but at the end of the day, your reaction to external and internal factors determines whether or not you succeed.

Accepting total responsibility for your weight-loss success and for the journey to reach that success also means abandoning the *fix me* attitude. Losing weight and improving your health becomes dependent on your actions, not on external factors or assistance. And you have the power and the ability to do it. You just don't have to do it alone. Let me be clear on this: You are not alone on this journey. You can find terrific support members, psychologists, doctors, dietitians, even medically supervised weight-loss centers. And you have this guide, a proven road map for success. Use some of them; use all of them; use whatever *helps* you get to where you want to be.

COLD FEET

Once you've made the decision to change, don't be surprised if you experience a few qualms or cold feet. This is natural. Most people worry about making changes, even when those changes are positive, healthy choices for a better life.

One of the chief concerns I hear from people embarking on a weight-loss program is about what they'll look like as they move through the program. It's all too true that beauty really is in the eye of the beholder. That said, people will notice changes to your physical appearance. Most people who observe the changes you're making are going to have positive responses. They're going to see you with a trimmer waistline and notice the way you carry yourself with greater confidence. They're going to notice that you're not carrying the extra weight in all the places weight so often likes to accumulate, that your clothes fit better, and that you're happier. In short, they're going to notice that you're taking steps to becoming a thinner, healthier you. The vast majority of people interpret weight loss and a thinner appearance favorably and conclude that it reflects better health and a better sense of well-being.

But not everyone will see it that way. Some people will notice that, as you lose weight, your skin loses the taut appearance it has had in the past.

For some people, extra weight gives the skin a more youthful appearance because the excess fat underneath the skin stretches the skin and makes it smoother. With the loss of a lot of that excess fat, the artificial smoothness of the skin is also lost and, because there has been excess skin stretched to cover the fat, losing weight can cause wrinkles. Wrinkles are often viewed negatively and associated with aging. So one potential risk, so to speak, or side effect, of weight loss can be a body that's at a healthier weight but that features a few more wrinkles. In my view, this falls into the category of a *good* problem to have.

Whether it's on your face or on your body, skin has to stretch to cover the fat underneath it, and it doesn't automatically shrink back once the underlying fat is lost. But excess skin isn't going to lower your quality of life, and it isn't life threatening. If it bothers you, there are steps you can take to reduce or eliminate the excess skin, including cosmetic procedures.

Try this exercise:

Calculate your BMI. You can use the formula here or the BMI chart found in Appendix B.

BMI is calculated using the following formula:

[Weight (pounds)] / [height (inches)]^2 x 703

Example: weight = 150 pounds; height = 65 inches

Calculations:
[150 / (65)^2] x 703 = 24.96

or:
[150 / (65 x 65)] x 703 = 24.96

or:
150 / 4,225 x 703 = 24.96

But, really, in light of the positive effects of losing weight, excess skin and a few wrinkles are minor.

The definition of insanity is doing the same thing over and over and expecting different results.

~ Albert Einstein

In order to make changes, you have to work through some challenges and learn new things. Not doing so and trying to tell yourself you're content with the status quo is inertia or self-deception. You probably can continue doing things the way you always have. For a while. But what you've been doing is destructive and unhealthy. Your body knows this already. It's just marking time before it makes its displeasure known, if it hasn't already.

I don't believe there are any true benefits to staying in the same place and not doing the work to lose the weight and become fitter and healthier. Because you *do* have the power to make these changes and to transform your life and because the data in favor of doing so is so very compelling, I see no reason not to.

Never talk defeat. Use words like hope, belief, faith, victory.

~ Norman Vincent Peale

2

.
.
.

Commitment

Earlier I asked you to take a few minutes and imagine what it would be like if you were never again overweight. I asked you to imagine your life; the things you'd do; the ways your life would be improved; the ways your friends and family would react to the new, healthier person I'm positive you have the ability to become.

Now I'm asking you to *believe* in that vision and to commit to becoming that person. One of the first steps to losing weight and keeping it off forever is learning to believe in yourself. There's no way to commit to something you don't think is possible. You may be able to fake it–stick to a diet; grudgingly exercise–but, until you believe in your ability to change and your right to a better life, you will inevitably slide back to old habits.

BELIEF

Take a moment to think back over your life. Think about all the changes you've made successfully. Did you graduate high school, go to college, find a job, raise children, and find love? Did you move out of your parents' house? Did you learn to drive? Take a road trip or fly in a plane? Have you ever ended an unhealthy relationship or taken the risk to pursue a healthy one? Have you worked for a promotion? All of these are changes you made because you believed they were possible. Hard as they were, or even as easy as they seemed, you would have never accomplished any of them if you'd thought they couldn't be done.

If doubts creep in, and they will, take a look at some of the success stories in this book. The people quoted herein are normal people with the same skills and tools available to you. They've shared their success stories to help you get to a place where you have a success story to share as well.

You can foster belief in yourself by visualizing and imagining the things you want in your life as if you already have them. But, believe it or not, belief takes practice. Those people who believe in themselves and rise to the top of their professions–from movie stars to athletes to CEOs of multinational corporations–practiced believing that they could do it. And they followed through on their belief in themselves.

> *You must begin to think of yourself as becoming the person you want to be.*
>
> ~ David Viscott

Focusing on your goals–visualizing them, committing to them, and believing in your ability to achieve them–can launch you into the steps you need to take to succeed.

In short–what you imagine, and believe, you can become.

FEAR

It's not always easy to ignore the negative thoughts that creep into our heads. Fear fuels those thoughts, and fear is a powerful enemy. It's hard to move forward when you're afraid that whatever you have and love in your life can be taken away if you make a change, but, really, that's just fear talking.

Take a look at some of the common fears people experience when embarking on a quest to change themselves; do any of these sound familiar?

- My skin will look old and wrinkly if I lose weight.
- I'll have excess, sagging skin if I lose weight.
- My friends won't like me if I'm not identified as a *fat person.*
- My spouse will get angry if I garner attention from the opposite sex.
- People are impressed by my successes; they won't feel the same if I'm not fat. They'll expect more, and I don't know that I can produce more.
- What if I lose the weight and I'm still not happy?
- What if I can't lose the weight after all?

Irv: A gold medal is a wonderful thing. But if you're not enough without one, you'll never be enough with one.

Derice: Hey, coach—how will I know if I'm enough?

Irv: When you cross that finish line tomorrow, you'll know.
                                                                ~ Cool Runnings

All of these concerns are based in fear. And fear only exists until we confront whatever has caused it. Someone standing on the edge of a cliff is afraid of falling, but that person is not falling. There's no proof that there will be any falling. And the person who does fall off the cliff is not afraid of falling; that person is worried about landing.

A gem cannot be polished without friction, nor a man perfected without trials.

~ Chinese proverb

The important thing, as I see it, is to get to the place where you *are* facing the challenges of how your partner and other people will treat you and how you'll feel about yourself if your skin looks wrinkly. Because when you're at the point of actually having to face those problems, it means you've lost the weight. But worrying about them before you even start losing weight is just fear talking.

Your goals are too important to be derailed by fears that don't help you. Placed in the context of your entire life, almost nothing you can do will have as positive an impact on your life, your health, your quality of life, your longevity, and, probably, your relationships as losing weight. What possible objections could justify abandoning such an important quest? Take stock of these negative thoughts and learn to ignore them.

Your future depends on it.

Courage is not the lack of fear. It is acting in spite of it.

~ Mark Twain

EFFECTIVE DECISION MAKING

There are lots of decisions in life—even big decisions—that you can make passively. For instance, maybe you take your vacation in the same spot every year because you love that place or because that's where your family has traditionally gone. Maybe you're following the preferences of a spouse or kids or other family members. This is a passive decision that doesn't require a lot of hard thinking. There's nothing wrong with doing what's worked before, but there may be other choices you're missing because you're comfortable with the old. Your vacation time could be spent in a thousand other ways—some better; some worse. You won't know until you actively consider your options.

Passive decision making works fine for many decisions in life, but some decisions, such as the decision to lose weight and keep it off or the decision to improve your health and your quality of life, need to be active decisions. These decisions need to be based on soul searching, on goal setting, and on really taking an honest look at yourself and asking what you want to achieve and who you want to be.

Too many of us never get to the point of making active decisions about our weight because, consciously or unconsciously, we just don't think we are worthy of anything better than what we already have. This is the worst possible form of decision making—the kind we don't even realize we're engaging in.

You may delay, but time will not.

~ Benjamin Franklin

The very act of making the decision to change is the first step in changing. By choosing to lose weight and put your health first, you're making a positive decision, but you may still need to convince yourself—and possibly others in your life—that the work is going to be worth it.

Effective decision making requires information and comes from the evaluation of all available options. Just as you have hundreds of diets to choose from, you have different routes you can take to achieve your weight loss. You can choose from a bewildering and wonderful array of physical activity—the sky's the limit—and the more fit you become, the more choices you'll have. You can choose to change your diet all at once or in increments. You can choose to pursue a low-calorie diet or a liquid protein meal-replacement shake regimen for initial weight loss. You can choose to leap onto another fad diet bandwagon and hope you end up looking like the celebrity endorser. The choices are all yours. But before you do any jumping, take time to determine which way you're jumping and evaluate which of your options will work best for you.

HUMAN BEHAVIOR

Just because you're doing something that will undoubtedly improve your life doesn't mean it will be easy. Most people on a weight-loss journey have specific consistent challenges. For some it might be family; for others it could be a busy schedule; still others may just be locked into old ways of thinking. And some of us may go along just fine until we hit a stressor, trigger, or challenge.

Family

There may be resistance from your family to seeing you change simply because change can be threatening. They may not understand you're becoming a stronger, healthier person and simply see you moving away from them. But forewarned is forearmed.

Take a look at the pressures against change in your life. If your entire family is overweight—or even if some members of your family are at normal weights or are underweight—and they simply love to eat, you have some challenges before you even start. Even if family members aren't actively working against you and even if they want you to succeed, certain behaviors—afternoon popcorn, Friday night pizza, Saturday morning buffet, Sunday morning brunch, celebrations in which food plays a major role, and on and on—can negatively affect your success.

If your family members are apt to feel threatened, what can you do to reassure them before you even start and once you're actively changing?

Time

If time is your nemesis and you're always running late, what can you do to ensure you're eating healthy on the run? Brainstorming ahead of time can reduce the impact of these challenges. Maybe you're fine when you have time to cook meals at home, but a late business meeting leaves you ordering from a snack machine. Perhaps you could make and freeze a few easy-to-reheat meals at home each weekend and bring them into work each Monday as a sort of "just in case" backup. If you don't end up needing that meal during the week, then great, that's one less meal you need to cook on the weekend.

Or maybe you don't have time to cook breakfast despite your best intentions. There's no reason to keep trying to force yourself to change the way you use your morning time. Instead, keep nutrition bars in a bag in your car or get in the habit of making a meal-replacement shake at night that you can just grab it and go in the morning.

The key here is to plan ahead. Don't wait until you're hungry and short on time to figure out what to eat. This is one of the foremost issues that I see daily in my practice.

> Make a quick list of circumstances that tend to put a wrench in your plans for healthy eating. Take that a step further now and brainstorm some ways you might confront those wrenches.

Stress

Your relationship with food, your planning, your habits, your thoughts, and your desires affect your eating and exercising behavior. Most of us know that stress can trigger eating, smoking, drinking, or other bad behavior. Stress management is vital to long-term weight management.

Learning how to vent, manage, or deflect stress will improve every facet of your life. Adding these new skills to your game plan can dramatically decrease the chances that you will go back to old, unhealthy habits.

Exercise is an excellent stress reducer. You may have been successful in the past at controlling stress with stress management strategies on your own, in groups, or through counseling or medical therapies. You should continue these sources of help until you've found a long-term stress management method that works as part of your everyday life. When you're confronted with stressful events, return to the principles that worked best for you. If those principles no longer work, don't give up. Go back to effective decision making, look at your options, and find new methods to control this insidious saboteur.

What are some stress relievers you've already found in your life? These could be anything from yoga to driving, deep breathing, reading, walking, talking to a friend (which is great to do on a walk, as it enables you to get exercise and stress relief at the same time), cleaning, gardening, doing volunteer work, or playing with a pet or child. What makes you happy no matter how hard your day has been?

Triggers

Triggers can be anything from circumstances to memories, events to destructive trains of thought, sights, smells, tastes, emotions–your list is as unique as you are. But no matter what the form, triggers enable old, destructive habits and behaviors. Learn what your triggers are and you can work to avoid the negative consequences they lead toward. For example, if going out to the movies always leads to eating a huge bucket of popcorn, anticipate the trigger (the great smell of buttered popcorn and the anticipation of the movie) and plan ahead for a different response (perhaps by bringing along a healthy snack to nibble on and a diet soda).

Take a moment to list the triggers you are aware of in your life. What circumstances have led you to go off your diet or exercise routine in the past? Which might cause trouble for you in the future?

Eating Out

Once you've made the decision to move forward with a weight-loss pro-gram—whether it's something you've put together yourself, you're working with a physician, or you've joined a weight-loss group or program—you're going to make significant changes to your lifestyle. Your eating habits will change, your diet will change, and your levels of physical activity will change as you pack exercise into a life that, in our day and age, I assume is already pretty busy. That's a lot of change all at once! It's all positive change, but even positive change can be difficult for normal, human, pat-tern-seeking minds to cope with.

So it might be a good idea to ease into the program you've chosen and go with it for a while before you start adding external challenges. There are going to be challenges already, whether they're in the form of professional lunches or a family that isn't joining you in your life-changing adventure. You might want to give yourself some time before you take on additional challenges, such as going out to eat with your friends.

On the other hand, you may not want to turn your friends down for every activity and abandon your social life entirely. So can you still enjoy going out for drinks after work or meeting your friends in a restaurant? This might be a challenge you're looking at with a great deal of trepida-tion, and you might be afraid that one evening out could be all it takes to trigger the beginning of the end for your weight loss. It can be scary to go to a bar or a restaurant and be surrounded by food and other temptations. Can you do that and stay strong?

Yes, you can, especially if you do some advance planning. Although, at the outset, it wouldn't hurt to suggest alternate activities, when the time comes that you do decide to go ahead and meet your friends for drinks or dinner, activate your creativity and visualize the exact results you want from the event.

One thing I highly recommend: If you're following a liquid-protein diet or some other form of meal replacement plan, stick to it. Take your shake or bar with you and have that. If you must chew on something, see if carrots or some steamed broccoli or cauliflower are on the menu and have that with a zero-calorie beverage. May I suggest that you even call ahead to check; don't wait until you get to the restaurant to discover that there is nothing but appetizers of the deep-fried variety. Remember, you're going out for the camaraderie, not the food.

Visualize the positive things you'll tell your friends when they ask questions and the comebacks you'll have for friends who might just tease and push a little. Prepare answers for friends who urge you to celebrate just this once.

Here are some of the things my patients' friends have said, as well as possible responses to them.

- You've been working so hard and look so good. Why can't you just enjoy tonight?
  Possible comeback: Because I really like the way I feel when I stick to my commitment to improve my health.
- What's the point of living if you can't have things that taste good/can't have things you like?
  Possible comeback: I have plenty of things that taste great, but I love the feeling that comes with losing weight and becoming healthier.
- You're looking a little pale/thin/under the weather. You should eat more!
  Possible comeback: I did eat more. Now I am working hard to become healthier, and I could really use your support.

I'm not suggesting that all your friends are intentionally trying to sabotage your efforts. But they're your friends. They want you to be happy. Food used to make you happy, and they don't understand (yet) the ways in which you've changed. If you and your friends have always enjoyed food and drink together, your friends may feel that, without your participation, the event is not as enjoyable. You just need to show them you're still you–just a leaner, healthier you–and that you can still have fun with them.

However, overweight friends who have relied on your overindulgences or unhealthy choices of the past to excuse their own can resent the fact that they now have no one to blame but themselves for their own behavior. And friends who are at normal weights may not understand the amount of effort, perseverance, and guts it's taking you to go after your goals or the amount of damage that can be done if you let go *just this once*. Since you know how much work you're doing to achieve your goals, you're forewarned and forearmed, in this case.

You also need to guard against the restaurant's intentions. Restaurants are in the business of selling food and, while they're not actively working against you and your weight-loss goals, they can present serious challenges. Keep in mind:

1. Many restaurants serve enormous portions. Even those that serve so-called normal portions almost certainly provide more food than you really need. Before you even order, have in mind that you're not going to finish the entire meal. Rather than worrying that you're wasting money or food, remind yourself that the alternative is to waste all the work you've been doing. (One alternative to feeling you're wasting food is to split a dish with someone else.)

2. Add it up ahead of time. Before you go out, take a look at your calories for the day. If it's a planned excursion, you might cut calories before going out.

3. Order only from the salad menu, though be mindful–in some restaurants, the salads can pack a worse caloric punch than the entrees.

4. Ask for salad dressing on the side. That way, you can control the amount you use.

5. Skip dessert or agree to split one with another diner, but just have a bite or two.

6. Focus on your dining companions rather than on your food. But when you're eating, pay attention to each bite. If you savor your food, you eat more slowly. Eating more slowly allows you to feel when you're getting full by allowing the satiety mechanisms to keep pace with your eating.

7. Keep bread, chips, and other appetizers on the far side of the table or, if you're sharing a meal with like-minded companions, don't have them at all. These *extras* are responsible for a large number of calories you really can skip.

8. Avoid alcohol, which has a good many empty calories. It also makes it easier to forget mindfulness and increases the likelihood of eating inappropriately. One glass of red wine is good for your heart and health, but any more than that is not.

9. Plan ahead. Brainstorm the potential challenges to eating out. Restaurant meals are often social events, and not everyone you're eating with will share your ideas on managing what you're eating. Visualize yourself staying on track and beating down temptations. (Remember, you can always have a healthy salad or a meal replacement bar or shake prior to going out. This will make things much easier when you are out and faced with all the choices.)

10. Enlist the help of a support person who can help you make healthy food choices and encourage you to stay on your plan if it looks like you're going to slip.

We never repent of having eaten too little.

~ Thomas Jefferson

GOALS

Before you can hit a goal, you have to know what that goal is. If you're vague about it, your results will be inconclusive. If you simply state that you want to lose weight, how will you know when you've reached the weight that's right for you? State your goals clearly and up front, whether you want to lose a certain number of pounds, hit a healthy goal weight, improve medical conditions, or eradicate diseases that have been complicated by your weight.

Defining your weight-loss goals is one important step, but I want you to take it another step further. I want you to chart a path of personal success that springs from your success in losing weight.

Start by writing your goals down. A goal that's not clearly stated is a goal that's easy to miss. You might want to travel more, get a better job, or lose weight, but if you never state your goals, clarify them, or make a game plan, you're left not quite ready to head to Ireland or become a vice president in your company or lose that 50 pounds. Until your goals are clearly articulated, it's hard to see the path you need to take to get to them. Once you've stated them, it's hard *not* to start on the road to success.

Shoot for the moon. Even if you miss, you will land among the stars.

~ Les Brown

Because the goal of losing weight is so important, I'm going to ask you to define it clearly in your mind. Then write it down.

Here are some of the specifics I want you to consider:

How many pounds do I want to lose?

What weight would I consider healthy for me?

At what weight would I feel proud, energetic, and confident about my abilities?

What weight would allow me to be more active, feel more attractive, date with confidence, or just accept compliments and know that the person giving them means them?

Do you have a number in mind? Good. Write it down. Then write down some additional goals as well. Be specific and let your imagination range. Have you always wanted to run a 10k race but found that it was beyond your ability? Have you always wanted to go skiing with your family at a favorite resort? Do you simply want to travel with more ease and less pain? Think about the activities your weight is keeping you from and write down the specific activities you want to pursue. Set goals for yourself that show specific, demonstrable activities and achievements.

Thoughts lead on to purposes; purposes go forth in action; actions form habits; habits decide character; and character fixes our destiny.

~ Tryon Edwards

Small Steps

At the outset of any major undertaking, there are going to be qualms. Running a marathon. Pursuing a graduate degree. Losing 100 pounds.

Oh, I could never lose 100 pounds.

Sure you could. Not in one day. Not in a month, even. But you *can* lose 100 pounds, and you can probably do it within one to two years. That's one to two pounds a week. Or you could lose five pounds a year over the next 20 years, for a total of 100 pounds.

With any major undertaking, one of the difficulties in moving forward is not being overwhelmed by the enormity of what you're doing. When the transcontinental railroad was imagined as a great unifying system for a broad and growing country, the vision gave many people a great sense of purpose. But, in order to actually construct the railroad and bring the vision to reality, many, many small tasks were required. It was the job of a great many engineers and surveyors and railway men to break down the mighty project into many small, manageable steps.

Now, your project of losing weight should seem like a more manageable project than creating the transcontinental railroad, and it is!

You don't have to see the whole staircase;
just take the first step.
~ Martin Luther King Jr.

So, your mission: to imagine this great project of losing the weight and becoming healthier as a series of many, small but manageable steps. Break the project down into manageable weekly chunks. Here's how:
- Make an appointment with your doctor
- Begin a committed Induction phase of your weight-loss program (see chapter 6) in order to lose weight more rapidly at the outset (this is important, as it provides the motivation that's needed to continue)

- Measure your body composition and body fat percentage (it's not all about what the scale says–the ultimate goal is to have adequate amounts of lean body mass and a healthy amount of body fat)
- Set your goal weights for the first month, three months, six months, and one year
- Write down your temptations, failures, and triggers as they appear
- Find a great psychologist to help you strategize ways to overcome the temptations and triggers
  - Establish weekly weigh-ins and find people to whom you are accountable
- Track your calorie intake (this is much easier than it sounds, provided you have a good calorie tracker)
  - Begin a plan of increased physical activity

Future Goals

Life never stands still. Time moves forward, even if you yourself are standing still. So I'll let you in on a little secret about goals: Once they're accomplished, they no longer seem so huge. And once they're accomplished, no matter how much you wanted them or how hard you worked to achieve them, you can feel a bit let down. You set a goal, you struggled, you persevered, you worked hard, and you won. Now that you're there–the "there" that seemed so mythical when you set out–what's next?

The more things change, the more they remain ...
insane.
~ *Over the Hedge*

Life never stands still. Achieving and maintaining your goals of health and healthy weight requires innovation and new techniques year after year after year. New goals will help you to maintain that weight loss and to keep striving to either stay at your new, healthy weight or continue moving forward until you reach it. Weight doesn't stand still any more than life does, and just because you win a battle, it doesn't mean the war is over.

Think forward, plan ahead, and adopt new strategies throughout the years. Keep your excitement engaged and always have something you're reaching for. Once you reach a goal, celebrate, cheer, tell the people you love–and then set another goal. One that's a little higher. A little harder. A little more challenging. (But one that's still, ultimately, attainable.) And with weight loss, I want you to adopt one new strategy or set one new goal right now and then set another six months from now, halfway through the year. That way, you'll be adopting two new strategies–creating two new healthy weight maintenance habits–every year.

Some of your goals are bound to fall away. Some of your strategies will stop working. Just as the healthy deli sandwiches will change or the running route will suddenly be under construction or your workout buddy will move away, other things will change as well. But so will your mind-set. You've been there and done that with regard to one goal or strategy. But when there's a new one–look out, because there's no stopping you.

Life has no limitations except the ones you make.

~ Les Brown

MEDICALLY BASED PROGRAMS

I think of an effective weight-loss program as being broken into at least three phases: the first being an *Induction* phase that sparks rapid weight loss (induction simply means inducing or initiating; in this case, initiating weight loss), a *Transition* phase in the middle, where you lose the rest of the weight, and a *Maintenance* phase after you've lost the weight so you can successfully keep it off.

Medically supervised programs work well because they bring a medical perspective to individual weight-loss efforts,and they can find conditions that may be blowing your efforts. In a *medically supervised* program, you're working to lose weight under the watchful eye of a professional who is deeply familiar with the unique health problems that stem from being overweight. The concepts in this book in this book are taken from the real-world experience of the medically supervised program at the International Metabolic Institute, also known as iMetabolic.

With a medically based program, you benefit from the expertise and guidance of many professionals who can help you on your journey. You'll ideally work with a physician, an exercise coach, and, possibly, a life coach, a dietary expert, and a psychologist, all of whom are focused on helping you achieve your goals. In addition, the best programs will have set up support groups where you can meet with other people who are going through the same things you are, exchange information, celebrate successes, and, perhaps, make new friends–friends who are definitely going to understand everything you're going through.

You can do this on your own, to a large degree, by taking advantage of the principles of a medically based program and the principles described in this book and seeking out other professional and support systems as you go.

Whether you are following an established program or winging it on your own, remember that you are unique and that your circumstances are unique. Your eating habits and preferences are formed out of your own experiences, including your:

- Food preferences
- Culture
- Medical history
- Physical activity level
- Work life
- Daily routine

It just makes sense to use each and every tool necessary to create a unique program tailored to your needs so you can succeed.

I encourage you to work with your doctor or with a medically supervised weight loss program if one is available to you. Look for a program that takes into account more than your weight and BMI; a program that puts your mind, as well as your body, into the equation; a program that is made specifically for you. Use this book as a supplement to that program. If you can't find a good program near you—one that brings together all the pieces of the puzzle—please use this book as the guide to the components you need to include.

· ·

For the last several years I've been bothered by my slowly increasing weight. Every time I tried to exercise and eat right, I'd lose a few pounds here and there, only to gain it right back.

The weight was taking its toll. My low back was bothering me, I couldn't bend over to tie my shoes, my clothes were getting uncomfortable, and my kids and wife were making fun of my big "behind."

As an anesthesiologist, I care for many of Dr. Sasse's bariatric patients in the operating room. Over the years, I've heard many of them speak about their successful pre-op weight loss using the bariatric shakes and the weight-loss program. I knew the shakes worked; I just needed some commitment.

With the program described in this book, I've been successful in losing 35 pounds. After going through the program, I found there were four keys to my personal success.

The first was the encouragement from my family. I have three children in their teens and early 20s, and I wanted to stay active and healthy because we do so much together as a family. Second was replacing what I used to eat with the meals and bars. My weight loss started during the first few days, and hunger was not really a problem. For me, it is impossible to just reduce my intake of regular food. Meal replacement was key.

Third was making a written commitment at iMetabolic and weekly weights. I needed to feel I was accountable to someone, even if, in reality, I was only accountable to myself.

Fourth was a concerted effort to be diligent about going to the gym. This took practice and focus. I needed to make it a habit before it even began to work.

For me, the program was a great jump start to helping me feel better physically. Now I'm really looking forward to this summer's boating season!

Kevin Lasko, MD—lost 34 pounds and 13.4 inches in 12 weeks

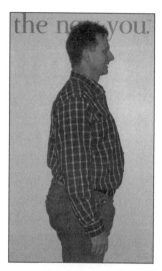
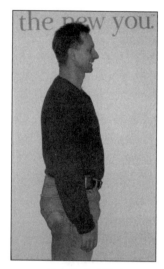

Kevin Lasko [Before] *Kevin Lasko [After]*

Weight-Loss Medications

Prescription weight-loss medications can play a helpful role for some people. As a group, the medications are very safe, with very few side effects. But they also offer only very modestly enhanced weight loss, which is usually not enough to get excited about. They are not a magic answer, but they can help some people–a bit.

A person whose BMI is between 18 and 25 is considered to be in the healthy range; a person with a BMI of 25 to 30 is considered overweight. Specialist physicians (like those in the American Society of Bariatric Physicians) recommend that people with BMIs of more than 30 consider adding prescription weight-loss medications to their weight-loss programs. Medication is also recommended for those people with a BMI of 27 or more who are already suffering from conditions brought on by being overweight, such as diabetes, sleep apnea, elevated blood pressure, and high cholesterol and other medical conditions. (See www.sasseguide.com for a comprehensive list of health conditions related to weight gain.)

Of course, your first concern when taking any drug, in addition to whether or not it will work for you, should be whether or not that medication is safe. In the wake of Fen-Phen, which made national news and caused harmful heart valve problems, it's sensible to ask a physician who knows and understands weight loss about the safety of these medications before ever considering starting a prescription weight-loss medication regimen.

Most weight-loss medications that are currently prescribed by physicians have been around for decades and have a long record of accomplishment of safety and common use, and medical studies have shown their effectiveness and supported their safety track records. While I'm going to touch on the side effects that are possible from each medication, I have to say that, in general, the currently available medications are extremely safe. The fact that these medicines must be prescribed by a physician and include monitoring and oversight increases their safety. A word of caution, however: Do not simply order these drugs (or any drug) from some source you find on the Internet. You never know what you'll get, and the costs to your health can quickly outweigh any savings you might have enjoyed.

Weight-loss medications aren't a magic bullet, and they're not going to provide long-term weight loss for you if you don't commit to your weight-loss program. The weight loss seen with these medications is modest—usually 5 to 15 pounds over a year as part of a weight-loss program—but every pound counts.

Phentermine is a mild stimulant that's about as powerful as a cup of coffee. It's been around a number of years, long enough that no drug company is making it under a proprietary name any longer; the medication is now sold as a generic and is not under patent. What this means for you is both that the drug has a long history and has been thoroughly tested and that its cost is much lower than it originally was.

Phentermine raises the metabolism slightly and suppresses appetite. It is one of the more effective weight-loss medications out there and it has the fewest side effects of any on the market today. When combined with a medical weight loss-program, phentermine results in slightly greater short-term and long-term weight loss.

Phentermine is usually introduced into a weight-loss regimen early—when the patient is moving from the Induction phase of the program to its Transition phase (see chapters 6 and 7).

Phentermine has few side effects. In some people, the stimulant effect can raise blood pressure, but that doesn't mean people who already have high blood pressure can't use the medication effectively; it simply means it's something a doctor is going to keep an eye on. Phentermine can also cause some mild stimulation or an increased sense of energy, but it's a very mild stimulant, comparable to caffeine, and most people build a tolerance to the effect fairly quickly. In some people, the medication can also cause insomnia or irritability, but both symptoms generally pass quickly. If the symptoms are a bother, the person can stop taking it.

Phentermine has sometimes caused a rash in people, but this is extremely rare, occurring in fewer than one in 1,000 people using the medication, as does constipation, difficulty urinating, and dry mouth.

In the field of weight loss, we consider phentermine to be one of the safest weight-loss medications on the market. If you're wondering, then, why you've never heard of it, the most likely explanation is that it was developed at a time when weight loss was considered a cosmetic concern rather than a serious health issue, so the FDA wanted the drug to be used very sparingly–for three weeks at most–and it was difficult to get a prescription for it. Most experts in the field, however, believe that the health risks from being overweight far outweigh the risks of taking phentermine.

Diethylpropion is a lot like phentermine, but phentermine is a once-a-day medication that works for approximately 20 hours, and diethylpropion has a shorter half-life. The benefits of using the medication, however, include the fact that it can be used to target specific times of day when a person is feeling the most need to control appetite. Otherwise, diethylpropion is very similar to phentermine, with the same very low risk of side effects.

Sibutramine (under the trade name Meridia®) is still under patent. It works on the neurochemistry of the brain, creating its effects through the neurotransmitter serotonin. While Meridia® does produce some modest weight loss when used within the context of a medically supervised weight-loss program, it's expensive and, in my opinion, is not as effective as phentermine. It does have a role in treating depression, and it may serve to help with both mood and weight problems.

Orlistat (which goes by the trade name Xenical® and, more recently, Alli®, which is the same drug at half the prescription dose and is sold over the counter) works by inhibiting an enzyme that works to break down fat in the digestive system. This causes the body to pass fats directly through the digestive system without absorbing them. This may cause the side effect of diarrhea. Another possible side effect is the loss of some fat-soluble vitamins. Most of us in this field consider orlistat to be very minimally effective, though occasionally it is prescribed for people who are suffering from constipation as the result of a high-protein diet.

Ephedrine and phendimetrazine both have effects and side effects that are very similar to those of phentermine, as well as other effects that your doctor might feel would be beneficial in your specific weight-loss program.

Topiramate has been successfully used in controlling binge eating and cravings. Often the medication can be taken just at night, and at fairly low dosages. While the dosage may need to be increased over time, the drug can be very effective in combination with a medically supervised weight-loss program and in combination with phentermine or another medication.

SUPPORT

One of the most valuable additions to your program is something that requires no professional degrees or special training whatsoever: a support group. Some, but not all, medically supervised programs offer support groups that you can join. If you don't have an established program available to you, feel free to start your own. The easiest way is to simply post a sign at work noting that you want to form a Saturday morning walking group with others who are in a program and striving to lose weight. Bingo–there's your support group.

You didn't get here on your own–you got here in part because of the pressures of life, because of the incredible availability of fast food and calorie-heavy foods, and because of the society we live in and the advertising around us. Family, friends, and the culture you live in have played a role.

In our society, food is often equated with good times spent with family and friends; it's entirely possible that the people you love the most contributed to your weight gain. If they're in the same place you are, your decision may help all of them to decide to lose weight, as well. But even if you're the only one, now is the time for others to play a part in helping you to restore your health.

In a good medically based program, you'll learn how to incorporate dietary changes, behavior modification, more physical activity, and other skills you'll need to make all these changes permanent. But one of the most important facets of a medically based program is the very fact that you don't have to do it all alone.

How often does losing weight seem overwhelming or impossible? Sure, you really can gain 20 pounds in only two or three weeks of bingeing and not working out, but it rarely comes off that fast, and it doesn't stay off if it does. So when you're looking at losing 30, 40, 50, or more pounds, you know that it's a challenging undertaking that stretches out ahead of you, and while there are plenty of diet books, they don't always agree, leaving you with questions that go unanswered and techniques that don't work. You need a proven system that focuses on you and that lays out a clear path to success.

Once you start with a program, you'll have a dietary plan that you've helped to create—one that takes into account your eating habits and your strengths and weaknesses and that is designed for you to get maximum weight-loss results while still getting the nutrition you need. Your dietary plan will take into account whether you're going to use meal-replacement protein shakes and bars or stick with a limited food plan. It will help you balance your eating and give you a list of suggested beverages and guidelines as to how much to drink.

Your medically supervised plan will also detail physical activity guidelines, because exercise will be an important component of the program. Even those people who aren't overweight benefit from regular exercise, so learning how to do it right and finding out what you love to do is important–exercise is something you're going to be incorporating into your life long-term.

Support Groups

You have the power to make a completely new group of friends to support you in your weight-loss journey. This doesn't mean you're leaving the others behind–it just means you're adding more people to your life; people with the same goals and dreams as yours.

If you've decided that your weight-loss program is going to involve formal medical supervision, you may find a support group (or several of them) already set up through that program. This is a benefit you really want to take complete advantage of. Support groups appeal to the social beings inside us. People are social creatures who like to share the highs and lows of life, celebrate successes, and have someone to commiserate with when things don't go as planned. In our society, a lot of those celebrations and commiserations involve unhealthy food. It's nice to have a group of friends for whom social interaction isn't dependent on food, and a support group can provide that setting.

Losing weight is hard. Keeping it off long-term is hard. You really need people you can celebrate the right way with, in ways that don't involve food. And there are going to be low moments, missed goals, and times when it all seems pointless or you're depressed, and what you used to turn to in order to feel better–a comfort food; a favorite restaurant meal–is no longer available to you. At those times, a support group can really help. These are people who can share what worked for them when they were right where you are. These are people who can honestly say, "I know *exactly* what you're going through," and really mean it.

Losing weight can get a little bit easier if you have people around to talk to who are pursuing the same goals and going through the same celebrations and disappointments. A support group can help you through low moments and be there to celebrate high times.

Putting Together Your Own Group

If you're not enrolled in a formal program and can't find a support group in your area, put together your own support group made up of your most supportive friends and family members. These may be people who have already taken journeys like yours or people who have dealt with other health issues. These are the friends who are always there for you or the family members with the most self-control (which they're willing to share when yours is low.) Tell them your goals of losing weight and ask for their support. Enlist a friend or group of friends you can call when you're feeling down or when willpower has ebbed and temptation has grown. Everyone has moments of backsliding, forgetting, or eating something out of habit and then feeling guilty. An amazing month of working out, eating right, and losing weight can be undone in one unplanned, unanticipated, and uncontrolled binge. From there, it's easy to just give up altogether.

Don't. Don't give up. Find the friends and family who can make up your support system and cheer you on. Keep their contact information close and your determination to call them when you need to closer. A friend's concerned, thoughtful response could stand between you and serious backsliding and lost time.

Surround Yourself with Winners and Losers

Weight loss and weight gain are contagious. OK, I'm a doctor, and I can't say they're medically contagious, but the behaviors certainly are *catching*. If you've ever been around a friend who has embarked on a healthy, positive, new direction in his or her life, you know that your friend is busy talking about all the new things that he or she is doing and is truly excited. It's the same thing with losing weight and following a new program that's already looking successful.

If your friends are at normal weights or have already begun to shed excess pounds, that's positive, too. These friends probably have healthier habits than you do. They think about food less and eat healthier when they do eat. Not to mention that studies have actually proven that, if your friends are successfully losing weight or are at normal weights already, your odds of becoming healthier and more fit and then maintaining that weight loss go up. The reverse is also true. If your dearest friends are overweight or obese, you'll find it harder to achieve your goals unless they are trying to lose weight too.

I'm not suggesting you abandon everyone in your life who isn't in perfect shape or that you go out of your way to cultivate a completely new circle of friends for no other reason than to lose weight. If your friends are overweight, your new determination can help them make changes that can, in turn, catapult your determination even higher. Tell your friends about your plans. Encourage them to encourage you. If you're all moving in the same direction and that direction is weight loss and improved health, you have a better chance of everyone achieving success. But your first concern is your own success—and, when it comes to sticking with friends who may not be supportive or helpful, at least know that forewarned is forearmed.

Try this exercise:

Calculate the average weight of your five closest friends.

START BEING THE HEALTHY NEW YOU NOW

When you make the commitment to lose weight, you make the commitment to change your life for the better.

When you actively work to lose weight, you actively work to change your life to a new and better one.

What you're doing in losing your extra weight is much, much more than simply seeing the numbers on the bathroom scale tripping ever lower.

Make no mistake about it; you're changing your life. You're taking control and you're making changes for the better.

Start making those changes today.

> *Our life is what our thoughts make it.*
>
> ~ Dale Carnegie

There are many ways you can start living as if you've already lost the weight. Start incorporating these changes into your day-to-day activities.

Physical Activity

Maybe you don't yet have the endurance and the fitness level that you're going to attain when you've lost that extra weight, but there's nothing stopping you from being active now. Take a brisk walk or go for a simple hike–whatever pushes you just a bit from where you are now. You'll be surprised how fast your cardiovascular fitness improves. For most people, it's only a matter of days before they find that their ability to exercise has increased markedly.

As you begin to exercise, hold your head high. Take pride in the changes you're making and start thinking as if you are already that fit, healthy person you aspire to be. Imagine yourself as that healthy, fit person who does this every day. Exercise isn't a chore; it's who you are.

Professional Life

The way you're perceived at work and in your professional life has a lot to do with how you carry yourself, the confidence you exude, and the way you speak, dress, and interact with others. It's true that being overweight is often a detriment when it comes to professional interactions. Overweight people are often perceived as less serious, less capable, and less accomplished in the eyes of colleagues. Yet you can overcome all of these biases by acting like the substantial, accomplished person you are with confidence and gravitas. Look people directly in the eyes. Speak with confidence, a smile, and a sense of humor, and you will go far.

Social Activities

Many people who are overweight feel embarrassed or less confident in social situations because of the extra weight. They feel that people are making fun of them or making comments behind their backs, or that others just don't view them as serious and capable since they can't even control their own weight. Many times conscious or subconscious beliefs hold people back from interacting successfully in social situations. Don't let anything hold you back. Smile confidently, look everyone in the eye, ask about others more, and be generous, encouraging, gracious, and giving. That is you.

Eating

One of my patients commented to me recently that skinny people never order the double cheeseburger. That's right, they don't. They value their fitness and maintenance of their waistline and health above the enjoyment of a huge meal. And so do you.

Start acting like that skinny person. Think about what it feels like to be that person who maintains his or her figure and fitness, pays attention to every bite that's eaten, and judiciously enjoys only what that person really likes to eat. Set the bar high for the food you put in your body: make sure it is really good or don't bother. Even in your daily eating, you can make use of the powerful vision of the person inside you–the healthier, fitter person you're striving to become. You can change how you eat, and how you feel about eating, right now.

Try this exercise:

Close your eyes and imagine bumping into an old girlfriend or boyfriend from high school. Now imagine that same encounter, but visualize yourself having already lost the weight.

If this change to a fitter, skinnier, healthier person sounds good to you, then start changing today. Close your eyes and feel what it is like to be that confident person. Now start acting that way today. The sooner you embrace the new person you're becoming, the sooner you'll become that person.

> *We become what we think about.*
>
> ~ Earl Nightingale

If you've made the decision to start living your life *now* as if you've already lost the weight, I applaud your decision. You're already seeing how wonderful your new life will be when you can engage in activities with friends and family and have the ability to be more active, more comfortable, and, I know, happier. Start thinking of other areas of your life where you can apply the steps of Visualizing Change, Belief, Setting Goals, Responsibility, Commitment, and ACTION. Many people like to focus on one change at a time, but it's certainly not necessary.

3

.
.
.

Life-Changing Exercise

There's a limited amount of time in every day, and even if you have the best of intentions, it's possible for the things that are lowest on your list of *want to do* to fall down the list until there just might not be enough time to get them done. It's easier to feel, if not virtuous, then at least not hideously guilty, if at the end of the day, *you truly meant to exercise but ran out of time* rather than decided there were other things on the list that had more priority or you just didn't feel like it or just didn't get around to it.

If asked, I think many people would say they don't like exercise. Often exercise conjures up the idea of boring, pointless, repetitive, and possibly painful movement. If you're considerably overweight, it may be very un-comfortable or even seem embarrassing to walk into a gym or head outside to work out. Trying to keep an at-home schedule can be even harder–it's easy to have the hours fly by until you find you never quite got around to it.

But there are a couple of concerns to take into account here. For one thing, *exercise* is just a word. Replace it with *physical activity* if you like that better, or *purposeful movement*, or anything that doesn't make you feel you're going to be imitating a hamster on an exercise wheel. Exercise can be a walk around the block to see how the neighbor's roses are blooming or who hasn't shoveled off the driveway after the latest snowstorm. It can be a hike in the woods with the family or a pickup game of basketball. All exercise really means is sustained physical movement for a set period.

You have to stay in shape. My grandmother, she started walking five miles a day when she was 60. She's 97 today, and we don't know where the hell she is.

~ Ellen DeGeneres

Exercise is critical to the long-term success of any weight-loss effort. Whether you're following a medically based weight-loss program, working with a doctor or dietitian, or doing it on your own, exercise is going to be a key component of your weight loss. Many people find that exercise is the piece of the puzzle that brings everything together because diet alone isn't going to fix weight problems.

EXERCISE TIPS

Here are a few tips on keeping your exercise program going:

1. **Do a variety of activities you enjoy.** You don't have to go to a gym. You don't have to spend loads of money. You don't have to do it with anyone else, nor do you have to do it alone. You just have to *do* it. Shift your ideas from regimented exercise regimes to having a variety of activities you enjoy–walking; lifting; running; tennis; cycling; hiking; swimming; aerobics classes– so you can do something every day no matter what time of day you get to do it, what the weather's like, or whether or not your workout partner flakes out on you.

2. **Find a workout buddy.** It's easy to blow off the rules when they're from you to you. Who are you to tell you what to do? Plus you can probably find a way to justify not meeting your own expectations. Letting someone else down is harder, especially if your workout buddy's instructed not to let you off the hook. Pick someone reliable and dependable and be accountable to each other. But don't let that person's schedule, choices, excuses, or lack of enthusiasm sabotage your routine.

3. **Make your workout a priority.** If you find something you love, it may start feeling like a luxury rather than a requirement—at which point, it may be harder to make yourself go do it when everything else is pressing. But exercise needs to be non-negotiable. You really can't ever *make up* a missed workout. Family, friends and coworkers are going to have to learn to accept your physical activity as a new part of your identity. (And who knows–they might even want to join you.)

4. **Exercise first thing in the morning.** It's a great way to start your day with the feeling of a job well done already, and it's a great way to avoid all those good intentions that don't quite pan out or having someone or something sabotage your best efforts. If you're going to a gym, find one located between your home and your work–that will get you on your way even quicker and, if you did think about skipping, you'd be passing right by it.

5. **Exercise on your way home from work.** It's the next best thing to first thing in the morning. And, if you don't go home first, you stand a much better chance of ending up wherever you meant to exercise–yoga class, the gym, that great walking trail–than if you try to go home, change, and go back out.

6. **Exercise even when you're too tired.** You'll be surprised how often working out will energize you, and you'll feel proud of yourself, to boot. If you really think you can't, just go to your workout site and promise yourself you'll do the absolute minimum. Chances are you'll do a lot more than that.

7. **Log your activity.** Nothing breeds success like success. Write down the facts that are important to you–how far you walked or ran or cycled; what you weighed; how it felt; distances; repetitions; what the days were like. The more entries you see on your workout calendar, the more you won't want to miss a day. (If you're walking, take a pedometer and count your steps. You'll be impressed at how quickly they add up and how short a time it will be before you're seeing what on-foot errands you can add to your day just to get more steps.)

8. **Notice every sign of progress.** Exercise is about more than just losing weight and fitting into a smaller size of clothes. It also means working out longer, having better endurance, going farther, and enjoying what you're doing more. Some of the many indicators that your exercise is paying off are:
    *   Getting a good night's sleep
    *   Thinking more clearly
    *   Having more energy
    *   Realizing your muscles aren't screaming after you've moved furniture
    *   Seeing your resting heart rate drop over time
    *   Hearing your doctor congratulate you on improved cholesterol, blood pressure, blood sugar, bone density, and triglycerides

9. **Compete.** Are you a competitive person, or do you keep that tiger tamed and inside? Exercise has a funny way of turning into something that calls for a bit of healthy competition, especially

with yourself. Don't shy away from it. Embrace the chance to strive for improved times, even if it is just around the block. Aim for completing a run-walk 5k if you have never raced or run before. Then think about how you can improve your performance and set higher goals.

10. **Reward yourself.** Sure, you should be exercising anyway, but if you are and you had to change your behavior to get here, acknowledge it! Making behavior changes is hard. Rewards motivate. So choose a goal–weight; distance; accomplishment–that has to do with your chosen exercise and go after it. When you achieve it, find a reward that works for you. It might be a new gym membership or new walking shoes, or it might be accessories for the new outfit you can fit into now. Pay yourself a dollar a workout, and your reward may even pay for itself. Do what works for you–and give yourself the praise you deserve for working toward it.

EXERCISE AS HABIT

Everything's easier once it becomes a habit (except habits you want to break.) Try walking every day for a week at the same time of day, then skip a day and see if you don't notice that something seems "off." You may find yourself getting restless or anxious or just plain missing it. But then, it's often not hard to start a new exercise program. Most of us have done it more than once. It might be complicated and full of bells and whistles such as exercise DVDs, gym memberships, or other people, or it might be as simple as heading out your front door every day to take a walk. It's easy to start.

What's harder is to keep going when the going gets tough. All too often, your initial enthusiasm and energy meet up with the reality of cloudy days or days after late nights, or you get a cold and take some time off and that lost ground seems too much to make up. It happens–energy wanes or there are other things going on in your life or you're not seeing results quickly enough–and you throw in the towel.

Set yourself up for long-term success. Make it fun. Pair it with other things you love, like listening to music, watching sports, spending time with friends, training your dogs, or exploring the outdoors. I'll share one secret with you: the harder you make it, the harder it is. In other words, if you like to work out alone and you force yourself to go to the gym with others, you're headed for trouble. On the contrary, if you thrive on companionship but think that all your training has to be solo and serious, you're setting yourself up to fail. Here's another secret for you: you don't have to hate it in order for it to be exercise. You can do something you *like* that's physical and that gets you moving–and if you do that, you're a lot more apt to stick with it.

A recent study by researcher Diane Klein, PhD, shed some light on the secrets of long-term exercisers who had been working out for an average of 13 years. Asked to rank what motivated them, their answers (ranked from most important to least) were:

- Fitness
- Feelings of well-being
- More energy
- Enjoyment of the exercise
- Making exercise a priority
- Sleeping better
- Feeling alert
- Being relaxed
- Weight management
- Appearance

And here's another secret: If you stick with it, it becomes addictive–in a positive way–more so than any food you ever craved. After a while, you begin to feel you could never live without exercise. And you can't.

3 • LIFE-CHANGING EXERCISE

LEAN MUSCLE

When you exercise, you don't just lose weight and rearrange where the weight sits and how it looks. Exercise actually builds lean muscle mass rather than fat. Lean muscle mass is what performs work and burns calories, so the more lean muscle mass you have, the better equipped you are to be a lean, mean, calorie-burning machine. For example, if, at the start of a diet and exercise program, you had 27 pounds of lean mass, your body could burn 1,300 calories every day without you doing anything. All you would have to do is sit and breathe and you would burn 1,300 calories. That'd be pretty nice. Now, say you spent a few months exercising and dieting and lost 10 pounds of fat while increasing your muscle mass by 5 percent–that would give you an extra 1.4 pounds of lean muscle mass, which would mean that, in that same day of calorie burning where you were doing nothing extra, you could now burn, say, 1,400 calories. By comparison, if you'd lost that entire 10 pounds by diet alone, you could have *lost* two pounds of lean muscle mass and eight pounds of fat, meaning you would have just lost a percentage of your at-rest, calorie-burning ability, and on those days you were doing nothing you would only burn 1,240 calories–and you would have gone through all that dieting only to find out you had less baseline, or at-rest weight-loss potential! That hardly seems fair, does it? Plus, we have to remember that five pounds of fat can be gained over the course of one year with as few as 50 calories per day that don't get burned. This just demonstrates how important the calories in, calories out relationship really is in terms of finding your body's calorie-neutral position.

If you continued to diet without adding in exercise, you would continue to lose lean mass, which means that, when you stopped dieting and started eating the same number of calories you were taking in before the diet, you would gain the weight back much more quickly. This syndrome does have a name, and you're probably familiar with it–yo-yo dieting. It's a version of what I call rebound weight gain.

So it's inevitable. If you want to succeed at losing weight and lose it for good, you need to add exercise into the mix. That doesn't mean you have to tackle the gym or even set foot in one. It doesn't mean you have to work out four hours a day or plant your flag on Mount Everest. You can start right this minute by doing something as simple as putting your shoes on and going for a walk around the block. When you come back from your walk, you will have achieved a number of things. You will have shaken yourself awake and changed your consciousness if you were drifting. And it's very likely that your mood will have picked up a little (exercise even stimulates hormonal changes that improve mood).

BONE DENSITY

What's more, exercise helps preserve the bone density in important areas of the body, like the spinal column and hips. Greater bone density means fewer fractures, a use-it-or-lose-it phenomenon that older people with thin bones know all too well.

HORMONES

Need some more convincing? Aerobic exercise, such as running on a treadmill, suppresses appetite, reduces the levels of the hunger hormone ghrelin, and raises the levels of the satiety (appetite-suppressing) hormone called peptide YY. So exercising can help you feel less hungry and, therefore, help you lose the fat!

In addition, you've just burned calories. It may not seem like a lot, especially if you only went around the block, but add up those same calories for daily walks over days, weeks, months, and years and you've got significant numbers. More important, perhaps, that walk you just took used your muscles, lungs, heart, and other organs in a productive, healthy way. You've taken steps (literally!) toward increasing your stamina and your cardiopulmonary function and, more important, you've increased your psychological sense of achievement and well-being.

The Multiplier Effect

Let's say you started walking around the block every evening. You would burn around 100 calories each time you did this. Now let's say you stuck with this for a whole year. A hundred calories per day multiplied by 365 days is 36,500 calories, which translates to 10 pounds lost per year–just by walking around the block each day.

BONES AND JOINTS

For people with serious orthopedic injuries or chronic wear-and-tear injuries to bones and joints, even that simple walk around the block is significant. If you have chronic injuries or if you're seriously overweight and putting stress on your joints with every step, start slowly and set achievable goals. Regular exercise, even mild exercise, does a world of good for your body and mind.

Take the first step, and your mind will mobilize all its forces to your aid. But the first essential is that you begin. Once the battle is started, all that is within and without you will come to your assistance.

~ Robert Collier

THE RIGHT EXERCISE

What sort of exercise should you do? The answer isn't the same for everyone. See Appendix C for some ideas. Choose something you love to do. If you can't think of any physical activity you love, start exploring. Try different activities until you find one you love. There's no surer way to fail at implementing an exercise routine into your life than by choosing something you hate. If morning is hell for you and being in a public place is unpleasant, then getting up early to head to the gym is going to be counterproductive. Conversely, if you feel awake and alive in the early evening, plan your activity for that time.

It's just as important to begin by doing something that you *can* do. Your exercise program has to be doable and achievable physically and mentally. If you have a serious physical problem that limits jarring movements to your axial spine, it's important that you don't take up a program of running on asphalt. Similarly, if you had a severe injury to your arms or shoulders, you might not want to start with racquet sports or other activities that could jar your arms and shoulders and aggravate the injury. This seems like common sense, but many people who don't want to work out in the first place may overlook such advice and sabotage their own efforts before they even get started.

Want some advice from others who have lost the weight and kept it off? The National Health Registry collects data on tens of thousands of such people. Want to know what the most common exercise is, as reported by these successful people? You guessed it. Walking.

For most people, starting off with something gentle, such as walking or swimming, can set them up for success. With respect to those mental expectations, don't be too ambitious. How many times have you or a friend gone out and bought exercise equipment or joined a health club, exercised vigorously the first time, and hurt so much afterward that you never went near it again? How many people around the country have dormant exercise machines collecting dust simply because the first few times they were used they caused so much discomfort or even injury? Don't get overly ambitious. You want to lose weight and get healthy, not scale a mountain or run a marathon. At least not yet.

What Do You Mean, *Take It Easy?*

If you're going to start by walking, it probably seems automatic to you. What is there to learn? You should be able to simply start. The reason your program will have guidelines in place is because you're going to be making so many other changes. If your weight-loss program includes a low-calorie diet (LCD) or meal-replacement foods such as shakes or bars, be especially careful to engage in only very low-intensity exercise activities, such as walking, until you have built up your strength and stamina.

We are what we repeatedly do. Excellence, then, is not an act, but a habit.

~ Aristotle

CONTINUING EXERCISE

So you've begun. That's an important baby step. Sleep well. Tomorrow, take another baby step and exercise again. And so on. It will be hard some days, easier some days, and *really, really* hard some days, so stay determined to take only the next baby step. You're changing your brain chemistry and changing who you are, and this takes time and repetition. Even if you get to the point where you feel guilty when you blow off your intended activity, it might sometimes seem easier to live with the guilt than to give up the time and energy to do the exercise. Don't give in: this is laziness in disguise, and it's your brain's attempt to revert to old patterns. Fight the old patterns and take that next baby step.

Once you get going with the exercise routine, and you're already passed that crucial 21 days it takes to create the seedling of a habit, then what? What if you take a couple of days off and feel tempted to never go back to it? Go back.

It's sometimes easier to muster the motivation to start an exercise routine than to stick with one–but, over time, sticking with it becomes your habit; your routine. In time, the baby steps become easier and exercising, just like commuting to work or feeding the dog, becomes something you don't even ponder. There are things you do, things you are and things you do that make you who you are. Exercise should be the latter.

Keep in mind that it's more than just the numbers on the scale or the fact that exercise is a part of your weight-loss program that keeps you going. Once you start, you're going to find other amazing benefits from working out, including:

- Feeling healthier
- Feeling more energetic
- Feeling less hungry
- Experiencing fewer headaches
- Lowered stress and improved tolerance of stress
- No more swollen ankles
- Better sex life
- No more aching hips and back
- Feeling ready to take on the world

A man's health can be judged by which he takes two at a time–pills or stairs.

~ Joan Welsh

4

.
.
.

Life-Changing Diet

"Diet" doesn't have to mean miserable deprivation. If you learn to eat well and to change your habits of eating, you won't have to spend every minute feeling hungry. What "diet" does mean is learning to eat in ways that are probably different from what you're used to. It means educating yourself in order to understand what foods are healthy and what foods aren't. Yes, you're going to be cutting calories and tracking how much you eat, and yes, you're going to be substituting healthy new foods for unhealthy old choices, but you're also going to be making sustainable changes and really understanding the forces of hunger and satisfaction that work inside your own body. Knowledge is power when it comes to food choices and weight loss, and knowledge gives you a lot of power when it comes to winning your weight-loss war.

Understanding what it is that you're putting into your body is essential. Once you know what it is that you're eating and drinking, you have the knowledge to make better decisions and take the right steps toward weight loss and attaining your healthy weight.

Reading labels and making conscious choices about what you're eating are an important step to lifelong weight maintenance. Over time, you'll see your daily choices add up. You're making choices about the foods you eat, the ways in which you cook them, and the number of calories you consume, and your body will change as you change these behaviors.

It doesn't take long to realize some obvious points, such as the fact that sweets and desserts are over-represented in most diets and don't provide enough nutrients to be worthwhile and that certain kinds of sauces, salad dressings, breads, pastas, and other foods routinely eaten at meals can have very high calorie contents, and that, if you don't think about it and eat mindfully, you're in danger of getting an overabundance of calories without enough nutrient punch. But once you have the information at hand, you can make healthier choices. Put your newfound information to work the next time you go grocery shopping. What do you have to lose? (Answer: the weight!)

To eat is a necessity, but to eat intelligently is an art.

~ Francois de la Rochefoucauld

UNDERSTANDING HUNGER

Hunger obviously plays a part in how much you eat and how much weight you gain. It's a basic human drive that should have been well studied by medical science by now and be well understood, but really, our understanding of hunger is fairly primitive.

What medical science does know includes facts about the specific regulators of hunger. We know, for example, that there are well-studied hormones that regulate appetite.

Hormones are chemicals secreted either in the brain itself or in the lining of the digestive track. Some of the most important include:
1. Cholecystokinin (CCK)
2. Pancreatic polypeptide
3. Peptide YY
4. Glucagon-like peptide-1 (GLP-1)
5. Oxyntomodulin
6. Ghrelin

The first five out of six of these cause us to feel full and make us want to stop eating. The sixth is a mixed regulatory hormone that, for the most part, increases hunger.

In classes on human physiology we learn that, when we eat, the stomach stretches and begins to dispatch some of the food down the intestinal stream. During that process, glands or secretory cells of the pancreas and the lining of the digestive tract around the first part of the small intestine secrete hormones in response to the food coming through. Some of these hormones are responsible for signaling the brain that you've had enough and should stop eating. Others cause the stomach to slow its emptying of food so the food is pulped further; this is the start of digestion.

Hunger is a signal to the brain that the body needs fuel. But we in the developed world long ago passed the time in history that we really needed this reminder in order to go find calories to consume. And there is no cutoff switch on hunger once you become overnourished and overweight.

Things can be messed up even further when you experience mental hunger. Hunger is more than just hormones and nerves and signals of an empty stomach. It can take place in your brain if you're expecting to eat at a certain time. You might still be full from lunch, but your brain signals it's time for dinner and convinces you you're hungry (thanks, brain). This is really just a kind of mental rut–you expect to eat because that's the time you usually eat. Since that is the time you usually eat, you must be hungry, right? And you must *need* food, right? Nope.

Another type of mental hunger comes from being bored, stressed, restless, or nervous–that kind of hunger can easily lead to grazing and constantly wandering in and out of the kitchen or break room as you search for something to take away the monotony.

Mental hunger can also be triggered by seeing food. If you crave one specific food and drive by the restaurant that offers it, your body can become convinced it's hungry. The same thing happens thanks to all that wonderful advertising out there. Those ads are slick, and their creators know just how to target them to create desires that you feel compelled to satisfy.

True hunger–the kind that comes when the body actually needs food–builds gradually and centers in the stomach, doesn't occur until several hours after a meal, and goes away once you've eaten. When physical hunger's needs are met, usually you feel satisfied. Some people, however, never really feel satisfied and keep right on feeling hungry. If you are one of those unlucky people and you have become overweight, you have to stop listening to hunger.

Emotional hunger comes out of nowhere, develops quickly, and is centered on taste–you crave something sweet, something salty, or a specific food (generally a snack or dessert food, not something healthy.) Emotional hunger can show up right after a meal, and it persists even when, intellectually, you understand that you don't need food. Instead of contributing to your well-being, the foods you eat because of emotional hunger can leave you wanting more and feeling guilty.

For someone who is seriously overweight, learning to live with some hunger is a good thing. Our brains and bodies might tell us they're hungry, but we don't have to listen to every word they say. Just because you're hungry before dinner is ready, that doesn't mean you can't wait the next hour until dinner is actually served. Satisfying that real hunger with a real meal at that point can be that much more satisfying.

When you feel hungry, stop and consider which hunger you're feeling. Drink a glass of water. Read a few pages of the book you're enjoying. A good walk could shake things up in a much healthier way. If you can't squeeze in a walk because you're at work, the weather is bad, or one of countless other reasons, find some way to distract yourself, chew sugarless gum, or have a zero-calorie beverage. It's hard enough to lose the weight and keep it of without turning to food for entertainment. Give yourself time to decide if it's emotional or physical hunger. Being aware of what's causing the hunger helps you determine the causes of emotional hunger. Being mindful of emotional hunger gives you control over what and when you *choose* to eat.

Try this exercise:

Write down your mental hunger triggers (such as boredom, stress, anxiety, depression, celebrations, and so forth). Now write down substitute behaviors for eating (things you can do to encourage weight loss rather than induce weight gain).

Success is not the key to happiness. Happiness is the key to success.

~ Albert Schweitzer

NUTRITION 101

If you want to succeed at losing weight and keeping it off forever, it's critical that you have an understanding of the basics of nutrition. Understanding what you're eating—and understanding the effects that food has on your body—are the building blocks of long-term weight-loss success.

They always say time changes things, but actually, you have to change them yourself.

~ Andy Warhol

With our caveman genes, we're eating in a modern world where a great deal of our food is engineered (cavemen had no perfectly shaped potato chips in their diets). In order to make the most of the food you eat and make the food you eat work *for* you and your weight-loss efforts rather than *against* you, you need to understand the components of what it is most of us are eating and drinking in today's world.

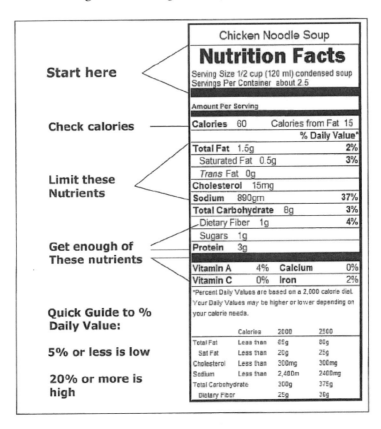

Note that the nutritional information is *per serving*. Most packaged foods contain more than one serving in a package. If you are eating more than one serving (which you probably shouldn't), you have to be sure you multiply the nutritional information by the number of servings you are eating. In the case of the chicken noodle soup depicted above, there is a total of 150 calories in the entire can.

Taking the extra minute or two to read the labels on the food you are considering purchasing can make the difference over the course of a week. Remember, you need to eliminate 3,500 calories from your weekly intake to lose one pound!

Try to select foods that are lower in carbohydrates and higher in protein. Once you start reading labels, you will be hooked. It will surprise you to see what some so-called *healthy* foods contain.

Reading labels is part of understanding what you're eating. It sounds simple, but there are tricks to reading and really understanding food labels. Almost every skinny person I know does read labels on packaged foods. But if you're buying something in a fast food or other kind of restaurant, it's a little harder. Some restaurants offer printed cards that spell out nutritional content so you have to make it a point to understand what you're reading. It helps to know the nutritional content of what you're about to eat before you eat it. This is, however, sometimes easier said than done. When you're in the grocery store buying food to cook or consume from a package, there's a label on that package, but others simply offer a Web site with that information, which isn't very helpful when you're trying to decide what to eat right then. One guideline, though, is this: if you're in a fast food restaurant to begin with, chances are what you're about to eat may not be very healthy fare.

Fast Food Order

You can immediately improve the probability that your meal will be healthier by *never* ordering a soft drink that has sugar or any calories, *never* ordering fries, and *never* "super sizing" anything, period. Figure out where the establishment you're frequenting posts the calories to every entrée and read up. You'll never order the same way again.

There are numerous reasons to read labels. You might want to check to make certain you're not eating or drinking anything you may be allergic to or to see if there are food additives or replacements you're trying to avoid. The main reason to read labels, however, is to know how many calories are in a serving. That's great information but, in order to make use of it, you need to know two things. What are calories? And what is considered a serving?

What Is a Calorie?

We talk about the energy contained in food by describing it in terms of calories. The term is so common that most people have stopped wondering what it means, exactly, and probably accept it as a unit for measuring what's in food or possibly for measuring food's effect on us.

That's not a bad start. A calorie is a measure of the amount of energy, or the heat, required to raise the temperature of one kilogram of water by one degree Celsius.

Sure, that helps. But what it means is that a physicist or chemist can measure the amount of heat required to heat a quantity of water one degree. That unit of energy is also used to describe every kind of energy we take in, whether it's something we drink or eat. (A calorie is actually a kilocalorie, a measure of 1,000 calories that are required to heat that quantity of water, but mostly we use a verbal shorthand and call the unit calories when talking about food.)

Every single person in the world has to take in calories in order to survive. Take in too many and you gain weight. Take in too few and you lose weight. Consistently take in too few and you can suffer from malnutrition or starvation. And for every single person out there, there's a level of caloric consumption that's, more or less, just right. It's the level of calories each person needs to supply his or her total daily energy expenditure (TDEE).

The TDEE is a combination of something called the basal metabolic rate (BMR) and the extra calories you expend during the day. Think of the basal metabolic rate as the minimum amount of energy, or calories, your body needs simply in order to exist and keep functioning at its baseline level (as if you were sleeping or resting all day). It means the amount of calories you need just to live–to keep your heart pumping and your body temperature regulated and your respiratory muscles working. Add your activities to the BMR and you have the total daily calories burned, or the TDEE.

This rate is a little bit different for everyone. The average TDEE for most adults in the United States is between 2,100 and 2,800 calories a day, with women needing calories on the low side of the scale and men needing more. The variations occur because of body size and composition. Men are generally larger than women and have a higher percentage of lean body mass. As mentioned earlier, the more lean body mass you have, the more calories you can burn at rest. An individual's BMR is not always obvious, but there are Web sites that can help you figure out yours. You can go to the iMetabolic Web site (www.iMetabolic.com) and take a look at the discussion on calculating your resting metabolic rate and what your general daily energy consumption is forecasted to be. Factors that affect the BMR include age, gender, percentage of lean body mass (muscle), and level of fitness.

One method of calculating BMR and TDEE is with an equation called the Mifflin–St. Jeor equation as follows:

BMR for Women:
10 x weight (kg) + 6.25 x height (cm)–5 x Age (yr) + 5
The answer is in units of kcal (calories) per day.

BMR for Men:
10 x weight (kg) + 6.25 x height (cm)–5 x Age (yr) - 161
The answer is in units of kcal (calories) per day.

To calculate the total daily energy expenditure (TDEE), multiply by an activity factor as follows:

Sedentary	BMR x 1.2 (little exercise)
Lightly active	BMR x 1.375 (light exercise)
Moderately active	BMR x 1.55 (moderate exercise)
Very active	BMR x 1.725 (hard exercise)
Extremely active	BMR x 1.9 (hard exercise daily)

You can take a body composition test, which will tell you your percentage of lean body mass and which can give you an estimate of your BMR based on your lean body mass level. Please be aware that this is only a forecast. As I've mentioned previously, BMRs can vary widely based on how an individual's particular metabolism is functioning. You can also take a more sophisticated type of test to measure your BMR in a doctor's office or lab.

Multiply your estimated BMR by your activity factor to get your TDEE; this is the number. Then multiply the BMR by your activity factor to give you the TDEE and this is the number of calories you must stay under, in daily food consumption, to lose weight over time.

Once you've determined what you need to stay exactly where you are weight-wise, you can start figuring out exactly how many calories you need to cut back on in order to lose weight. If you require 2,300 calories a day to stay exactly at your current weight and you cut back 500 calories a day, you'd lose roughly a pound a week. (Remember, 3,500 calories equals one pound.) Then add in what you could lose if you started exercising regularly and burning even more calories. There are Web sites that tell you how to figure out what you can lose with specific exercises over specific time periods. For example, if you burn an average of 370 calories in an hour of brisk walking, add that to the 500 calories a day that you've eliminated from your eating, and you are close to 1,000 calories a day. (That's nearly two pounds a week of weight loss right there.)

Knowing your basal metabolic rate and TDEE can be helpful, especially if you're trying to figure out why some people who eat more than you never gain a pound or why someone else is losing weight so much faster than you if you're both doing the same thing. It's very likely that the person who's losing so quickly has a higher percentage of lean body mass. This means that he or she can eat more calories because those calories are going to be burned off more efficiently. Remember that lean body mass is more demanding of calories than body fat.

Back to Those Labels

Remember that discussion about reading food labels? Here's why you need to make reading food labels a habit: By reading a food label, you can see exactly how many calories are in that food. If you have an idea of how many calories you need per day to survive and how many you need to cut out in order to lose weight, then, when you read that an item has 300 calories, you can make the decision as to whether or not this is a good use of your calorie allotment.

That's not the whole story, of course. A reasonably low-calorie food item that is nothing but carbs would still be a bad idea because it will have very poor satiety effect—it will leave you hungry for more in a short period of time. And, along with what it is you're considering eating and what its caloric content is, you're also going to want to take into account the serving size. This is one way food packagers try to get past the Food & Drug Administration requirements of listing the (often horrific) nutritional content of a package of food as a whole. How many times have you picked up what looked like a single-serving-sized package of potato chips, for example, and noticed that the packager has decided that there are two and a half servings in that little package? Trust me, they're hoping you're not going to do the math and figure out that you're not about to consume 200 calories worth of chips, but actually 500 (2.5 x 200 = 500)! Even if math isn't your strongest subject, it's not hard to see that you're actually getting a lot more calories than that modest number featured next to the words "per serving."

At which point you have a choice. You can consume the package of chips. You can consume one serving from it, thereby eating only the 200 calories you were anticipating. Or you can look hard at your decision and decide whether or not these potato chips are sublime enough to spend something like one quarter of your available calories for the day on them. Knowledge is power. Use it to your advantage!

Once you learn to read, you will be forever free.

~ Frederick Douglass

Making Use of Basal Metabolic Rate

One more way that knowing your basic rate of caloric consumption can help you is fairly basic and hard to argue with–essentially, if you need 2,500 calories to stay at the same weight during normal daily activities, you can take in 2,500 calories and lose weight if you increase your activity level to burn off additional calories.

If you need 2,300 calories to stay at the same weight during normal daily activities and you eat 500 calories more than you need every day, you'll gain roughly one pound every week.

If you need 2,300 calories to stay at the same weight during normal daily activities and you consistently make a point of eating 500 fewer calories every day, you'll lose roughly one pound every week.

It really is that simple, which is why understanding what calories are and what's in the food you're eating truly matters.

One Web site that allows you to calculate your estimated basal metabolic rate is at: www.calculator.org/bmr.aspx

---

There are simple ways to lose some of those calories, too. In addition to adding actual, intentional exercise to your days, you can make it a point to burn more calories whenever you can. One of my colleagues uses the stairs to come and go from his 10th-floor office. I'm not quite as dedicated as he is, but it's important to him to use the stairs whenever possible. You can use the stairs and eschew elevators and escalators. You can park farther away from the office, the grocery store, and even the gym in order to add steps to your day. Little efforts that you can assimilate into your life easily and quickly add up to make a difference.

What Food Is Made Of

Calories are an overall measure of the energy of food, but foods are made up of basic components. There are three basic components that give food its caloric energy: protein, carbohydrates, and fat. That's it—all food falls into one or more of those three categories—and, if you're reading labels carefully, you're going to see that, under the listing for the number of calories in a serving of food, there are listings of the grams of protein, carbohydrates, and fat in that serving of food. There may be other information as well, such as the amounts or percentages of minerals and vitamins in a serving of the food, but these are not. components that supply calories.

One of the reasons it's important to understand the breakdown of the components of food is that it will help you when there's not a lot of label information. It will also help you understand in detail what you're eating when there is label information.

The amount of each component of food–protein, fat, and carbohydrate–is listed in grams. Each gram of that component has a certain number of calories. For protein and carbohydrates, every gram produces four calories of energy. For fats, every gram produces nine calories of energy. A one-ounce chunk of cheddar cheese, for example, contains about eight grams of protein and nine or ten grams of fat. Eight grams of protein equals 32 calories. Nine grams of fat equals 81 calories. So your snack of a one-ounce piece of cheddar cheese–which is about the size of your thumb–weighs in at about 113 calories.

You can use the same formula for food products that don't generally come with food labels, such as meat–once you find out what an ounce of a certain cut of meat usually contains, you can understand that, for every ounce you're consuming, you're getting so many grams of fat and protein. Calculate those grams by the number of ounces you're having, and you know how many calories you're getting from that piece of meat.

Fats, with nine calories per gram, are the most energy-dense food source. It's one of the reasons that the first low-fat diets that sprang up focused on cutting out all fat; cut out 10 grams of fat and you've cut nearly 100 calories right there. As it turns out, however, cutting out all fat from a diet is not such a great idea.

Fat does do something good that carbs and protein do not do as well–fats create satiety, or satisfy our hunger. Humans tend to stop eating after we've had our fill of fats. Sugars and other carbohydrates, on the other hand, provide only a fleeting sense of satisfaction, and then a rather disturbing and unwelcome return of our hunger rather quickly.

Carbohydrates can be utilized as a rapidly available energy source, converted to glycogen (a stored energy source for the body to draw on quickly), or stored in the body's adipose tissue through a metabolic process called lipogenesis. The carbohydrates are converted and stored as lipids and fats in the liver, in subcutaneous fatty tissues, and in visceral fat tissues throughout the body. To put it simply, due to processes developed to support our need for energy when food might be scarce (hello, caveman

78

genes), extra calories from carbohydrates–in fact, extra calories from all sources–are stored as fat in the body.

The energy from fats tends to last longer and you get a more sustained energy from eating that piece of cheese than from something sugary or full of starch, which produces a fast peak of energy and dissipates quickly. Research has shown that carbohydrates may, in fact, be a more potent stimulus of the biochemical, metabolic processes that cause more hunger and more fat creation and storage. So knowing the breakdown of what you're eating can help you target foods that can help you create an energy deficit.

You can create an energy deficit–taking in fewer calories than you burn–by reading labels on the foods you eat and understanding the components that make up those foods. If you're looking at a product that packs a whopping punch of carbohydrates and almost nothing in the protein and fats realm, you're looking at eating something that's going to be stored primarily as fat and that won't provide much satisfaction or satiety. Keeping track of the components of the foods you eat can help you consume fewer, but healthier, calories throughout the day. Cutting your calories from more than you need or from your TDEE will help you lose weight.

Let us not be content to wait and see what will happen, but give us the determination to make the right things happen.

~ Peter Marshall

Increasingly, science is moving toward recognizing that real potent stimuli of insulin secretion isn't helpful or healthy–in other words, those spikes of energy from eating carbohydrates–the touted *sugar rush*–adversely affect your health by promoting an inflammatory state and atherosclerosis, or plaque buildup, in arteries.

Does that mean low-carb diets are finally getting the recognition they deserve? Maybe. What it does mean is that if you're looking to lose weight and cut back on high-calorie foods that aren't so good for you while eating more foods that are good for you, you're probably going to be looking at cutting back on carbohydrate consumption and increasing your lean protein consumption. In addition, since protein contains amino acids, and amino acids are the building blocks of muscle, protein can help you build and maintain your lean body mass, and the more lean body mass you have, the easier it will be for you to burn that fat you are trying to lose. It's nice the way that all fits together!

We've talked about reading food labels and about the importance of understanding how much you're consuming in the way of carbohydrates, fat, and protein. At this point, you may be thinking, *Fine; now I know about carbohydrates, protein, and fats—but I still don't know what any of those really mean.* Knowing the components that make up food and what they mean to you can give you a major leg up in your weight-loss efforts.

Carbohydrates

Carbohydrates are prevalent in all kinds of foods, from grains (such as oats) and wheat to sugars. When you're searching out carbs on a food package label, you'll be able to identify flours and grains easily enough, and all labels list the total number of carbohydrates in each serving of food. But if you're interested in breaking it down further and really understanding what you're eating, then you need to know that a good many carbohydrates have names that end in *ose*. The most common is sucrose—plain old table sugar.

Table sugar is actually a diglyceride, which you may actually see listed on the label among the ingredients. Diglycerides are made up of two different carbohydrates that are linked together (in the case of table sugar, glucose and fructose). Once you eat a product with diglycerides, your body will break down the sugars into individual components and will have two sugar molecules to store somewhere or burn as fuel.

In an interesting and alarming trend, consumption of sugar and other carbohydrates–especially sugar in the form of fructose, particularly high-fructose corn syrup (HFCS)–is skyrocketing now, both in the United States and around the world. If you were to plot the rise in sugar consumption over the last 30 to 40 years on one graph and plot the rise in obesity on another, you'd discover that these trends are very nearly parallel.

Fructose is consumed in massive quantities in the United States It's the primary sweetener in soft drinks and packaged desserts, and it also shows up in unexpected places, such as condiments. It was bad enough that prepared cakes used to be full of table sugar; now they're loaded with high-fructose corn syrup to make them taste even sweeter.

Our big appetite for sweets, along with U.S. farm policies that have favored corn production and consumption, have contributed to the alarming growth in consumption of high-fructose corn syrup. Most troubling is the close association between childhood consumption of HFCS and childhood obesity.

There's some evidence that fructose, and high-fructose corn syrup in particular, lead to greater enhancement of fat creation and fat storage and may increase insulin resistance, which is linked to metabolic syndrome (increased lipids in the bloodstream, increased blood pressure, and development of diabetes).

Not all carbohydrates are created equally evil. Most of the carbs you need to avoid or at least limit are refined, or simple, carbohydrates, which include white flour, table sugar, and high-fructose corn syrup. The more convenient and packaged a food, the more refining was done to it. Take oatmeal as an example: The old-fashioned (not instant) oatmeal that comes out of the big cardboard tube and is cooked on the stovetop is a healthy food that hasn't been overly processed. The oatmeal that comes in delightful flavors in individual servings and just needs boiling water poured over it has been heavily processed–giving it about the same nutritional value as you'd get from eating a Pop-Tart® (but don't do *that*, either.)

The traditional, non-instant, healthy oatmeal belongs to a class of carbohydrates called complex carbs, which have a different effect on the body than simple carbs. Complex carbohydrates are found in whole grains, vegetables, and legumes (such as peas and lentils) and, while they're still sugars or starches, the molecules of the foods have bonded together to form long chains that break down more slowly in the body, providing a longer release of energy while limiting the amount stored as fat. Because complex carbs break down more slowly, they don't cause the *sugar rush* effect of simple carbs or the rebound hunger that comes back so quickly with simple carbs. This is why even low-carb, low-calorie diets often include vegetables and why, when you reach the Transition phase of your plan, you'll see toast in your choices–this means whole grain, not white bread!

In today's world, we already consume far more carbohydrates than our bodies need. So, while the jury's still essentially out, there's more than enough evidence to suggest that high-fructose corn syrup is at least as harmful as other sugars–and that carbs in general aren't the best choice for energy if you're trying to lose weight.

Fats (Lipids)

Most people think of fat as either a solid, like butter, or as the fatty tissue found in chicken, beef, and other foods. Fat is actually composed of a number of different molecules, the core molecule being an essential fatty acid, or free fatty acid.

Free fatty acids are linked together in different chemical structures and stored throughout the body in different ways, including as fats and triglycerides.

Essential fatty acids are necessary to the body and must be consumed to replenish the body's stores. The most famous among them are the omega-3 fatty acids, which are predominantly found in fish oils. There are also omega-6 fatty acids, which are also known as linoleic fatty acids. These essential nutrients aren't produced by the body, so you need to get them from your diet, meaning you can't follow a diet that removes all fat and still be healthy. You need fats for the creation of certain molecules, hormones, and steroids that aid chemicals in the body in nerve signaling and for the creation of cell walls and membranes.

There's one other type of fat that you've almost certainly heard of, and the media played a big role in getting it out of most foods. Trans fatty acids are associated with hardening of the arteries and with malignancies, and the American Heart Association and the American Society of Bariatric Physicians, along with many other health organizations, have urged everyone to cut trans fat out of their diets. As a result, the FDA now requires food labeling to list exactly how much trans fat is present in any food. Knowing how bad trans fatty acids are and avoiding them in your food won't help you lose much weight, but it will keep you safer and healthier while you lose the weight.

The bottom line is that we need certain amounts of fat in our diet. And fats in foods give us a sense of satisfaction that just does not come from carbs or, to a lesser degree, even protein.

Protein

Protein is the last of the components of food. As in carbohydrates, there are four calories to every gram of protein. Protein is not stored in the body as readily as carbohydrates are, and it is essential for building muscle, which adds to your overall lean body mass and gives you greater fat-burning potential, even at rest. Protein also doesn't cause the same degree of insulin secretion and development of metabolic syndrome as carbohydrates do. Protein does not give us a "rush" of blood sugar followed by a craving for more.

Until recently, most experts assumed that all Americans consumed enough protein because American diets are traditionally rich in meats and dairy products. Some countries aren't as lucky. In sub-Saharan Africa, for example, many people develop edema and have large, swollen bellies due to a buildup of fluids that occurs as a result of lack of protein in the diet.

Until recently, the U.S. food pyramid and other sources recommended that something like 15 percent of your daily calories come from protein. Really, that's too low, and now most authorities on obesity and weight loss put the target (for those who do not suffer from diabetes) at around 30 percent. Most likely, what you should be shooting for is at least one gram of protein per kilogram (2.2 pounds) of body weight–so, if you weigh 150 pounds, you'll be looking at a minimum protein intake in the neighborhood of 70 grams per day which is 12 percent of the total calories if you're consuming 2,300 calories a day. Twelve percent is much more in line with recommendations for diabetics. Most of us who treat overweight patients and who have worked hard to learn the most successful methods for weight-loss success set a target of daily protein consumption of 100 grams or more for most overweight individuals. If you want to know what that adds up to in calories, multiply the number of grams by four. One hundred grams gives you 400 calories that you should be getting in the form of protein.

That's pretty reasonable, really, and protein generally tastes good. While it might not taste as good as chocolate cake or potato chips, protein in the form of cheese or cottage cheese, a good steak, or a nicely roasted chicken is satisfying. And diets that emphasize protein consumption–like the very famous diet espoused by Dr. Robert Atkins–generally feel more more satisfying and less like a sacrifice and are more sustainable than some other diets.

So are there any downsides to greater protein consumption, especially when recommendations are now going as high as 1.5 or 2 grams per kilogram of body weight? Someone suffering from kidney failure or renal insufficiency could have a hard time processing the protein. Protein is filtered through the bloodstream by the kidneys, so someone who's already experiencing stress on the kidneys could have trouble with the body's filtering system being overloaded. But such instances are fairly few and far between, and they're detectable via a routine blood test. (See Appendix E for more on sources of protein.)

Food is an important part of a balanced diet.

– Fran Lebowitz

Other Nutrients

Really, the only other nutrients out there are water, which has no actual nutrient value but is certainly important to health and survival; fiber, like cellulose, which isn't digested but aids in digestion; and micronutrients, like vitamins and minerals.

Vitamins have no calorie content, but they do contain molecules that play important roles in nutrition. Many vitamins are cofactors in chemical reactions that take place in the biochemistry of the body or in the metabolism. Some vitamins are already in great supply in our bodies; others need to be replenished on a regular basis. If they're not, the effects on the body can be disastrous.

For example, back when sailing ships were exploring the world, sailors who went for months without citrus or other sources of vitamin C learned firsthand that a lack of vitamin C in the diet causes scurvy, a disease that results in skin and neurological abnormalities.

Deficiencies in other vitamins and minerals can also produce disease states in the body. Another classic example involves iron. If the body doesn't get enough iron or if iron is depleted the body, as it can be in menstruating women and in people who have other conditions that cause chronic blood loss, the body can't manufacture new blood cells. A shortage in red blood cells results in anemia, which is a low blood count. Anemia causes fatigue and paleness and can present a real problem if it progresses and becomes more severe, though anemia can usually be resolved simply by getting enough iron in the diet.

Vitamins fall generally into two categories: water soluble and fat soluble. The fat-soluble vitamins are A, D, E, and K. Each has a different important role in the diet. Vitamin D has been getting a lot of attention in the media lately. It's associated with calcium metabolism, and vitamin D deficiency, which is more prevalent than was previously realized, leads to fatigue and loss of energy. Calcium deficiencies can lead to osteoporosis and may be associated with weight gain.

The water-soluble vitamins include most of the rest of the vitamins and the B complex, which is particularly important. Doctors often see vitamin B deficiencies in people who are seriously overweight, the most common being a deficiency in B_{12}, or cobalamin. Thiamine deficiency is also common. Both deficiencies can produce abnormalities of the nerves. People with B_{12} deficiencies can feel tingling or numbness in the hands or feet that can result in severe weakness of the extremities. Thiamine deficiencies tend to affect cognitive behaviors and cause problems with nerves, often in the form of tingling or nerve pain, which is called neuropathy.

These vitamins are not generally stored in the body, so it's important

---

We need sunlight to convert vitamin D to its active form. So people who live in cold climates and people who don't venture outdoors have higher rates of vitamin D deficiency.

---

to get enough of them through the foods we eat. In my opinion, with any weight-loss program where you're trying to create a calorie deficit and, ideally, are trying to emphasize proteins and cut carbs, it's important to take a multivitamin that includes both the water-soluble and fat-soluble vitamins as well as the important minerals, including iron. Vitamin B_{12} is a little different because it's not well absorbed when taken orally. It's usually given as an intramuscular injection, but today there is a sublingual variation that can be placed under the tongue and absorbed.

Alcohol

Alcohol is unique among the foods and beverages we eat and drink. Alcohol or ethanol is a unique two-carbon molecule that contains seven calories per gram. Sometimes you'll hear that you can drink while following a weight-loss plan because wine and beer aren't fattening. Actually, alcohol is a calorie-dense molecule, and if you continue to drink it, you'll continue to gain weight and store more calories as fat. The typical alcoholic beverage can contain anywhere from 100 to 300 or more calories in alcohol alone (and don't forget that there are probably more calories in whatever it's mixed with). The more you drink, the more wasted calories you consume–calories that have no nutritional value at all and that do nothing for you but raise your calorie consumption.

However, it's been clear for a long time that consuming a modest amount of alcohol probably has a favorable effect on our overall health (although heavy alcohol consumption clearly has a negative health effect). It's long been recognized that the people of France and other wine-consuming nations have lower blood pressure, lower lipid levels, and greater longevity than would be expected in such countries. This has been described as the *red wine paradox* and recently, some molecules (especially one called resveratrol) present in red wine have been associated with improvement of some health conditions, so it is likely true that moderate amounts of red wine (say, two to three ounces in the evening) do have some favorable effects. It's important to recognize, though, that we're discussing one small drink a day–more than that is probably going to have an adverse effect and shouldn't be consumed. Alcohol in more significant amounts can be associated with all kinds of adverse health conditions, including elevated blood pressure, liver disease, and weight gain. Moderation is very definitely the rule, and if moderation doesn't work for you, avoidance is the only answer. Your health is too important to not take care of it.

WHY DIETS DO AND DON'T WORK

Most people don't like diets any more than they like exercise. What's to like? Diets almost always involve deprivation and giving up the things you really like. Yet people make fortunes selling diet plans; and many people snap up each new plan that comes along whether it's logical or not; whether it's medically endorsed or just backed by a celebrity; whether or not it involves something alarming, such as eating nothing but cabbage for a few months. There's a whole section on diets in bookstores, and there are thousands of Web sites that promote specific diet plans and that allow you to sign on and chat with others who are following the same plan.

And the diets work. Of course they do. They wouldn't take off like wildfire across the country if they didn't. The problem is that every diet is going to stop working after a while because the discipline is impossible to maintain, you're too bored to continue following the same eating plan, you miss what you used to eat, or the plan is just plain too complicated. Try cutting all the carbohydrates or all the fat–or both!–out of your diet for very long and see what's left for you to eat.

How many of these popular diet plans
have you tried? Make a list.

- Atkins
- Optifast
- Low fat
- LA Weight Loss
- Weight Watchers
- NutriSystems®
- Zone
- Jenny Craig
- South Beach

In the beginning, you almost undoubtedly lose weight no matter what low-calorie plan you choose if you stick to it. But early success is typically followed by failure all too soon. How many times have you been on that roller coaster ride, telling yourself that, this time, it's going to stick?

Up to 95 percent of those who lose weight by dieting end up regaining that weight. Usually, dieters end up gaining back even more than they'd lost because they've lost lean body mass or muscle mass along with the fat.

4 • LIFE-CHANGING DIET

All happiness depends on a leisurely breakfast.

~ John Gunther

An eating plan that's based only on short-term deprivation or simple food selections doesn't work in the long run unless four critical pieces come together to make it a success:

- First, the calorie-restriction diet is carefully designed as an initial first step.
- Second, it includes generous amounts of protein, vitamins, and exercise–the key building blocks for creating more lean body mass.
- Third, it leads directly into the next phase of your comprehensive weight-loss program and doesn't just dump you off at the curb of rebound weight gain.
- Fourth, it is the action you take as a result of the inner life change you have made to become a leaner, fitter, healthier, and happier new you. The changes you need to make come from within you and build upon the knowledge gained and principles outlined in this book.

When you're looking for long-term weight-loss success, whether you're working with a medically supervised program or doing it on your own, you need to think past the concept of dieting as a short-term activity you'll do only until you hit your goal weight. Most people consider a diet anything but permanent. Whatever it is you're giving up today in order to fit into a special outfit or look good for a special occasion, you're already looking forward to eating those foods you've given up.

And that's not going to work–not in the long run–unless you make a commitment to change your life.

89

You don't need another diet plan that only works for a short while. You don't need to keep choosing among the diets hyped by movie stars on shows–diets that are designed in such a way that you regain the weight a couple of months after going off them. What you need is a road map to long-term success that's already worked for a great many people before you; a plan based on science and proven in the clinical setting of reputable weight-loss centers.

Try this exercise:

Calculate how many pounds you've gained each year for the past three years. If you don't change your diet and activity, how many pounds do you think you'll gain in the next three years?

By design, diets are non-sustainable; it's far better to view a diet as a prelude to long-term weight loss or as a jump start to success than as the entire journey in and of itself.

Precious little data shows any correlation between long-term success (beyond one year) and any of the popular diet programs. The concept of a very low-fat diet appeared to make sense, and its adherents claimed that such a diet reduces risk of heart disease and fatty atherosclerotic plaque. The low-carb pioneers made compelling arguments that diets low in carbohydrates are more sustainable and lead to greater weight loss with less rebound weight gain.

There's some truth to all of these claims. Think about it for a minute: You know that, at some level, the calories you take in must be balanced by the calories you burn. So, in a global sense, you must shoot for a reduced intake of calories, regardless of whether those calories come from carbs or protein or fat. Fat has nine calories per gram, far more than carbohydrates and protein (each of which has four calories per gram), so it makes sense to reduce some fat grams wherever possible, thereby cutting out a lot of calories.

But it doesn't end there–a calorie is not just a calorie. Carbohydrates cause some special responses in the bloodstream, starting with an abrupt rise in blood sugar. That leads to surges in the hormones insulin and leptin, which serve to lower blood sugar back to normal. (Fats and proteins do not produce this response.) As this repeats itself over and over, the body needs to keep raising the levels of insulin and leptin, like someone who needs to keep shouting louder to get his message across. In time, the cells become less able to hear this message (this is called *insulin resistance*), and this is the start of type 2 diabetes.

Perhaps the worst thing about carbs is that they leave us hungry again very quickly, and this leads to our eating more of them. Good for the makers of high-carb foods, maybe, but bad for the waistline.

No diet is the total answer. The answer. To get that, we need something much more profound and sustained.

Creating a Calorie Deficit

In order to start working to lose that weight, you're going to want to create a calorie deficit. That means nothing more than using up more calories than you're taking in. When you have a calorie deficit, you burn more calories than you consume.

Calorie deficit is simple. All you need to do is make sure that the total number of calories you consume in a 24-hour period are fewer than the total number of calories, or total amount of energy, you burn during that period.

The way in which calories are burned is broken down into two components. One component is the baseline, or basal energy, that your body burns via involuntary activity that keeps you alive, such as breathing and digesting food. The other component is the calories you burn through intentional activity, such as walking or exercising. Together, these two components comprise your total daily energy expenditure (TDEE).

Here's an example of the numbers: the average person needs somewhere around 2,500 calories a day just to balance the TDEE. Men generally need a few more and women a few less, maybe around 2,700 for men and 2,200 for women, but 2,500 is a good number to use as a general example.

Using the 2,500 calories needed for a typical day's activities, you want to increase your energy expenditure so that you're burning more calories through extra activity–extra exercise–and using up more calories than you're taking in.

Unfortunately, the scales are already tipped against you. Most people in today's society are already getting far more than 2,500 calories in a day and it's easily possible to get 1,500 to 2,000 calories in a simple fast-food lunch that doesn't even leave you satisfied. Not to mention that portion sizes have gotten bigger and that many of today's processed foods contain additives, such as high-fructose corn syrup, that increase calories without increasing the nutritional value of the food in any kind of healthy way. At the end of the day, it's easy to have consumed 3,000 calories without even knowing it. Consuming all those extra calories obviously results in weight gain.

With this diet, you're looking to create an energy deficit and the bigger the energy deficit–and the better the weight loss. For example, if you were to cut back 500 calories a day, you'd end up losing about one pound a week. That might not sound like much, but at the end of the year, you'd have lost over 50 pounds, and that is significant.

Cutting back 500 calories every day from what you usually eat, with no other changes, can result in the loss of one pound per week. Over the course of a year, that's over 50 pounds!

So, creating an energy deficit is an effective weight-loss strategy. It's also one that's hard to keep in place in the long run. That kind of long-term program is available with the help of a bariatric physician like me, a medical specialist who can help you fine-tune your program, offer insights into the health effects of such a diet strategy, and point out individual techniques and tools that might work better for you.

A fitness component is critical to the long-term effectiveness of any diet. By getting in more activity each day–taking more steps during the day, exercising, and so forth–you'll burn more calories and increase your daily calorie deficit.

Finally, there's the nutritional component. A number of studies have shown that to really successfully lose weight you need to decrease, dramatically energy consumption whereas probably the biggest keys to long-term weight management rely in large part on continuing regular exercise.

Change is the constant, the signal for rebirth,
the egg of the phoenix.
~ Christina Baldwin

Following is a list of medically based weight-loss concepts for successful life-changing weight loss. These concepts are based on science and on what has worked at iMetabolic, a comprehensive, state-of-the-art, medically supervised weight-loss center.

- Commit to changing your life.
- Follow the specific menus and program outlined.
- Pay attention to, and reduce, your caloric intake. Pay particular attention to reducing unnecessary fat calories.
- Focus on reducing carbohydrates. The sugar in our diets is increasingly recognized as the main culprit in obesity, increased hunger, and progression to diabetes.
- Exercise. Start, continue, and never stop.
- Modify the plan to maximize what works for you.

• •

I am a 66-year-old grandmother (I was 65 when I started the iMetabolic program). After more than 50 years of yo-yo dieting and after spending another miserable summer, I was determined to take charge of my life and live instead of just existing.

I saw the commercial for iMetabolic on TV and was drawn to it because this was a medical weight-loss program, and I'd never done that.

Of all the diets and weight-loss programs I've been on over the years, I've never reached my goal. I know I will here because kind and caring staff keep me wanting to succeed. I know there are many ways to enjoy my success.

Where there's a will, there's a way.

When I began, I had a lot of health issues:
   1. High blood pressure
   2). Scoliosis
   3. Polycystic ovaries

4. Diabetes
5. High cholesterol
6. Kidney disease

Even with these conditions, the nutritionists were able to work out a food plan for me. All I had to do was follow it and get as much exercise as I could. Weight loss was slow but steady, and I'm learning to keep it off. It's never too late!

*Sally Kwapich—lost 76.7 pounds and 46.15 inches; her BMI has gone from 40.6 to 28.1; she has become **non-diabetic**; her blood pressure medications have been cut in half; and lab tests show that her kidney nephropathy is improving.*

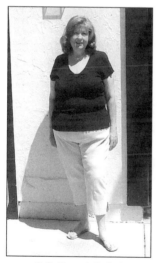

Sally Kwapich [Before]

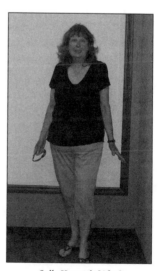

Sally Kwapich [After]

To be successful, a weight-loss program has to have a few critical features. Remember that you're trying to do more than fit into a bikini or look good for a specific event or watch the numbers on the scale drop. You're trying to achieve nothing less than long-term health improvement and improvement in your longevity and quality of life. You're changing your life, not following a three-month-long prescribed course of eating.

So, the diet you choose has to have the key feature of being sustainable; it has to be one that you can follow for a lifetime. Before we start on the specifics of the program, let's point out some key features of plans that fail and some key features of plans that succeed.

The Top 25 Reasons Why Diets Fail

But knowing *why* diets fail is an effective tool in your arsenal to fight weight challenges.

1. Having a negative or defeatist attitude.
2. Going on a diet that fails to phase in your stages of weight loss and weight maintenance.
3. Believing that you will eat low-calorie, monotonous fare every day for the rest of your life.
4. Letting the scale ruin your mood and letting a depressed mood affect your actions and your eating, for that matter.
5. Not drinking enough water (dehydration has many negative health consequences, and it can be interpreted by the body as hunger).
6. Drinking sugar-laden drinks, including fruit juice.
7. Consuming processed foods more often than fresh foods.
8. Not having an overall proven plan.
9. Not being aware of the nutritional benefits or detriments of what you eat.
10. Finishing every last bite of a meal, even after you're full.
11. Going back for seconds.
12. Skipping breakfast.
13. Starving all day, then bingeing (or eating something unhealthy just because it's "quick") at night.

14. Falling off the wagon, bingeing, and starting over tomorrow…
15. Thinking you are genetically destined to be *fat*.
16. Treating *fat* as a personality trait…
17. Not living each day to the fullest and believing that the "good stuff" will come only when you're thin.
18. Thinking that pills, powders, or potions are more powerful for weight loss than they really are.
19. Thinking of exercise (physical activity) as a chore instead of as a way to improve your weight, health, and life.
20. Indulging excessively in alcohol…
21. Watching sports rather than participating in them…
22. Watching too much television.
23. Thinking that dieting sprees, rather than lifestyle changes, will garner permanent weight-loss results.
24. Consuming fast foods on a regular basis.
25. Waiting for tomorrow to get started.

MAKING CALORIE REDUCTION EASIER

Calorie reduction is a big, vague concept. Here are some tips to help break it down into easier steps that you can take to meet your weight-loss goals.

1. **Zero-Calorie Beverages**

   Everything you drink should have zero calories. Eliminate all drinks that are sweetened with sugar, high-fructose corn syrup, or other calorie-laden sweeteners and replace them with beverages that are unsweetened or that contain calorie-free sweeteners such as Splenda® aspartame and stevia.

2. **Read Every Food Label**

   Know what you're putting into your body. Know the number of calories and grams of protein and carbohydrates per serving. Know how many grams of fat there are in everything you buy, eat, and drink. This alone will help you make smarter choices.

3. **Work Hard to Reduce Carbohydrate Intake**
   This means total avoidance of beverages that contain high-fructose corn syrup. Limit the turbo-charged desserts and snacks that contain huge amounts of carbohydrates. How will you know how many carbohydrates are in these things? Because you're reading every label, so you know the content of everything you're putting in your body.

4. **Avoid Excess Calorie Intake**
   Since you're following rule #1 and rule #2, this part will be easy. As you look at labels, multiply the grams of fat by nine (there are nine calories in every gram of fat) to get the number of calories of just fat in a serving so that you can recognize the true caloric cost of what you're planning to eat. You'll automatically begin limiting the fat in your diet.

5. **Exercise for Life**
   Exercise and diet go hand in hand. The calories you bring in and the calories you burn are the foundation of a plan for success.

SUSTAINABLE WEIGHT LOSS

The key to weight-loss success is long-term sustainability. In your heart, you know there are short-term changes you can make that will work–short term. You may be able to sprint a certain distance, but you can't maintain that speed for a marathon distance. The same is true for the monumental changes you make in your life–exercise regimens or diets or other activities you can take on for a certain period of time.

It's time to be honest with yourself and to make changes that are positive and sustainable. The changes don't have to be brutally hard. (Some of them, like giving up routine desserts or sugared sodas, might feel brutally hard in the beginning, but they won't for long.) But you have to commit to the changes you make, and you have to make them habits.

BRAIN CHEMISTRY

The first time you perform a new behavior, your brain isn't comfortable with it. Physically and mentally, you may be uncomfortable, but if it's something you want to do, you force your way through it. The next time you do it, it's a little easier. It's a little more familiar; the pathways in your brain have seen this pattern before. The third time, it's a little easier still. By the fourth, fifth, sixth, and one thousandth times, the path is well worn and the brain has become accustomed to the events that take place during that specific behavior.

Athletes who repeatedly compete at a high level, repeatedly perform their routines flawlessly, repeatedly visualize themselves winning gold medals–and, in fact, repeatedly win them–are much more apt to continue to repeat the habit of performing at that high level and will continue to win.

Choose a new behavior–maybe something as simple as forgoing dessert. If you've always asked for the dessert menu or asked the cook in your house, "What's for dessert?" skipping dessert will require building new habits. The first time you create the habit, ask yourself, "How am I going to get up from this table and move on with the evening without having dessert?" Then just do it. You might create a new ritual, like drinking a nice tall glass of ice water, to replace the old one of eating dessert.

Habit is habit and not to be flung out of the window by any man, but coaxed downstairs a step at a time.

~ Mark Twain

The first time you change your behavior, it's difficult. But the next time is a little easier. How many repetitions does it take before this becomes truly a sustainable habit you're unlikely to break? That's debatable, but it's probably in the neighborhood of at least several hundred repetitions. With each repetition, the change becomes less difficult. By the time you've repeated the behavior several hundred times, you probably won't even think about it.

Somewhere along the line of repeating your new behavior long enough to create a habit, you may relapse. This isn't failure. Beating something as ingrained as a lifelong destructive eating behavior is hard. Some people never backslide; others do several times before the new habit sticks. If you're one of the latter, and it takes more attempts, you should know that you're not a failure and that you are still going to succeed. You just need to muster the courage and determination to try again and to not give up.

Take care of your body. It's the only place you have to live.

~ Jim Rohn

The National Weight Control Registry uses data to follow people who have successfully lost and kept off weight. By examining people who have successfully lost weight and then maintained sustained weight loss, a few lessons have been learned.

What we've learned is that you don't have to be doing heroic acrobatics to stay healthy. You don't have to be running a triathlon every month. You don't have to be devoting four hours a day to vigorous exercise. What you do have to do is be steadfast in getting your exercise. The most common exercise reported by these people who have won big by losing weight in a sustained fashion is, you guessed it, walking. These people average 30 to 60 minutes per day of walking. Not hard. Very enjoyable. And it leads to all kinds of additional benefits, such as taking time for reflection and enjoying life. Stopping to smell the roses, as it were. If you're interested in taking a look at some of the stories of other people who have lost weight and kept it off–like you're going to–take a look at the National Weight

Control Registry's Web site (www.nwcr.ws). You can also share your own successes there as you go along. Current members have lost everything from 30 to 300 pounds and kept it off an average of 5.5 years. Nearly all of them modified food intake, and 94 percent increased physical activity on the road to weight loss.

Healthy Habits

Habits are nothing more than patterns of behavior you've fallen into. They're what you're used to. Habits can be ingrained on purpose–such as by creating new habits of exercising daily, reading labels on food packages, and weighing yourself at the same time every day or so. Habits can also come along on their own, of course–and often those are the ones referred to as bad habits. These include making unhealthy food choices, eating mindlessly, and sitting down to channel surf, without really watching anything or doing anything healthy in the process, at the same time each evening.

If you've battled your weight for a while, you've probably been overeating for some time. There can be a variety of reasons that a person can begin to overeat but, after a short time, it simply becomes habit–you're used to eating a certain amount, or you're used to having certain foods at every meal, like bread, or you've always had dessert and dinner doesn't feel complete without it.

> *Motivation is what gets you started.*
> *Habit is what keeps you going.*
> – Jim Ryun

These are habits, and not only have you probably already broken at least several of them, you can also establish your own habits to outsmart the part of you that wants to overeat at meals. To change what you're used in favor of what you want to become used to, you need to slow down and take a look at what your normal eating behaviors or habits are and, then find, ways to overcome those habits or behaviors. Here are a handful of tips to start the ball rolling:

- Make overeating difficult. Cook exactly the serving amounts you (and the people eating with you) expect to eat. If you have to make more in order to eat more, chances are you won't bother.
- Live with some hunger. It won't kill you; in fact, it will make you stronger and healthier.
- Serve in the kitchen. Only place plates of food on the table. If you're going to have seconds, at least you'll have to get up and walk over to get them.
- Keep the healthy foods—vegetables and fruits—available. Keep the unhealthy ones in a place that's hard to get to.
- If other people in your household are still eating foods you need to avoid, ask that those foods be kept out of sight (and out of mind). Hide them in the back of the refrigerator, freezer, or pantry. And definitely make certain they're in single-serving portions, just in case you do stumble across them when willpower is at a low ebb.
- Eat only one serving size (or less) of any food. Buy smaller packages of foods you don't really need in the first place, because the larger the package, the more you're going to eat. If you're buying from a warehouse club, repackage the contents of economy-sized packages to smaller containers when you get home.
- Eat from smaller plates. A healthy-sized serving on a smaller plate will look more satisfying than it will if it's lost on a jumbo-sized dinner plate.
- Eat only in the kitchen or dining room—not in the car; not while working; not while watching television. If you have to eat at your desk, stop working and pay attention while you eat. Make certain you're aware of what you're eating.
- Beware of leftovers. The more you have, the more you will feel

compelled to eat. (If you have leftovers, you made too much to begin with!) Dish out leftovers as you would any other meal and make certain of serving sizes.

- Forget about eating until you are *full*. Try to never feel full. Eat as little as you think you can get away with, then leave the table and move on with your day. You've had plenty.

Balancing Your Meals

You're constantly being told to eat a balanced meal. Occasionally, you may even hear that having a balanced meal eliminates the need to diet. But just what *is* a balanced meal?

Basically, half your plate of food should be vegetables and fruit. The other half should contain protein and starch or other carbs. That's it. Pretty simple, really. But what it does mean is that an entire plate of pasta isn't a balanced meal–clear half the pasta off the plate, add a steamed vegetable, and you're on your way.

MEAL-REPLACEMENT SHAKES AND BARS

Controlling calories is hard to do, especially when there are so many choices before you. When I'm helping a patient begin a high-intensity weight-loss program, it's nearly impossible to describe exactly how thin to slice the cheese to avoid extra calories or just which size of egg or strawberry counts for how much. Research has shown that eliminating all those choices and all that guesswork–and temptation–from the process of the initial Induction diet is far more successful. Replacing all those choices and temptations with a carefully controlled meal-replacement plan ensures that you get the right formula of calories, protein, vitamins, and the right mixture of amino acids, minerals, fats, and carbohydrates.

Lead me not into temptation. I can find the way myself.

~ Rita Mae Brown

Beyond that, using meal replacements works in the real world. And that's a huge advantage, since most people who are trying to lose weight are stuck living in the real world. I've seen success with meal replacements over and over again, and I use them myself as a technique to maintain a healthy weight. (Like many specialist physicians who direct medically supervised weight loss centers, I start my day with a protein meal-replacement shake or bar, and I usually have them as my morning and afternoon snacks, as well.)

Like most of the scientifically based, medically supervised weight-loss centers, ours recommends utilizing meal-replacement shakes and bars that are formulated with protein and the proper mix of nutrients that aid healthy weight loss. It takes food out of the equation. All of the choices, all of the decisions, and all of the temptations to sneak in a few extra calories here and there are simply eliminated. In addition, meal replacements provide an easy solution to not skipping meals, which can be very problematic from both a weight-loss perspective and a weight-maintenance perspective.

The shakes and bars accomplish several critically important goals. They:
- Provide a healthy protein source to build lean body mass
- Speed metabolism
- Eliminate temptation and the guesswork involved in trying to prepare just the right amounts of foods
- Suppress appetite
- Fulfill the modern-day practical needs of being tasty and convenient, and are therefore actually used successfully

5

.
.
.

The Plan to Change Your Life

You *can* lose weight. You *can* keep the weight off. Despite so many examples to the contrary, there really are a number of successful people who have lost the weight and kept it off for good.

Your long-term health success takes hard work and determination and a belief that you will succeed. It also takes a *plan.* Here's the outline of a simple plan that I have seen work for many, many different kinds of people:

1. Believe in yourself. You can do this.
2. Define your goals. Write them down. Be specific.
3. Personalize your plan to *you.* Pick exercises that you can actually do. Don't just wade into some atrocious diet and impossibly difficult exercise program. Set yourself up for success, not failure.
4. Begin. Even if it's not the perfect plan or the perfect program. Even if all the stars are not in perfect alignment. Begin.
5. Start with an Induction plan (see chapter 6). Hit it hard in the beginning. Be aggressive. Get the pounds off early.
   - Use meal-replacement shakes. Choose shakes that are high in protein and low in carbohydrates; you won't feel hungry and they won't push you to rebound weight gain.
   - Use your muscles. Increase your muscle activity every day, even if you're just taking a walk or using five-pound hand weights.

- Shoot for consuming no more than 1,000 calories a day initially.
- Weigh yourself every day.
- Make use of support groups.
- Take multivitamins and maintain your protein intake.
- Stick to this Induction plan–phase one of your weight-loss program–for 90 days or until you have lost your first major milestone goal weight of, say, 25 to 40 pounds.
- Set a target of losing 60 to 70 percent of your excess weight during the Induction program.

6. After your Induction phase, move to phase two of your weight-loss program: the Transition plan (see chapter 7). Start to slowly introduce some selected real foods and build upon good habits.
   - Emphasize protein first; eat everything else at your meal second if you still have room.
   - Make use of low-calorie, lower-carbohydrate, and prepared meals.
   - Stick with your exercise program.
   - Participate in support groups.
   - Weigh yourself every day.
   - Re-read your goals every day.
   - Create lifelong habits for successful weight maintenance.

7. Once you have finished the Transition phase of your weight-loss program, begin the Maintenance plan (see chapter 8) and make it a way of life.
   - Keep using protein shakes and bars for certain meals and snacks to reduce hunger and keep your daily calorie count low. A shake for breakfast and a shake or bar for each morning and afternoon snack seems to make sense for most people.
   - Continue to make sure you are taking in all of the protein and vitamins you need.
   - Think daily about *the multiplier effect:* the small things you do every day that, over the course of a year, can account for significant decreases (or increases) in your weight.

• Keep going with proven elements, at least periodically: daily weigh-ins, support groups, food journal, and use of prepared, low-carb meals, snacks, and shakes.

Your goals, minus your doubts, equal your reality.

~ Ralph Marston

Studies predict that by the year 2025, over 90 percent of Americans will be overweight or obese. Research shows that lower weights are healthier weights and that people with lower BMIs have longer life expectancies with less risk of cardiovascular disease and cancer. In this country, we're rapidly approaching the point at which nearly every person among us should lose a few pounds. But even if your goal is simply to maintain your current weight, a medically based weight-loss program has elements that work for you and your long-term goals.

The ideal weight-loss program is, of course, the one that works. The ideal weight-loss program is the one that succeeds in helping you reach your goals of losing weight and becoming healthier and more active; of becoming the person that you want to be.

But the ideal weight-loss program is not some external item that you pick up on the sales rack. It is a program in which you become heavily and completely invested. The ideal program, then, is one that appeals to you and works in sync with you and your habits, goals, and ways of living. For that reason, the ideal weight-loss program may not be exactly the same for every single person.

One of your challenges is finding or creating a program with the combination of nutrition, exercise, oversight, and expertise that works for you, but also one that challenges you. If there are aspects of the program that are deal breakers for you, that's different than if there are aspects that are challenging but that you can overcome. Look for a program you can jump into with both feet, even with its challenges. Look for a program that isn't so foreign to your way of life that you lose interest or can't overcome the challenges.

Let me give you an example. When Luke came to me as a patient, he was middle-aged and significantly overweight. He'd started gaining weight after college and never stopped. By the time I met him, his weight hovered in the range of 295 pounds. Worse, he'd fractured a small bone in his foot. The pain was severe, so any exercise routine that required Luke to put weight on that sore foot was doomed to failure before it even began.

I put Luke on a strict calorie-restriction program and got him started in psychological counseling and some sessions with a health coach. Those three components were accompanied by exercise that did not involve putting weight on his feet (such as work with light hand weights, swimming , and eventually, riding a stationary bike) proved successful for Luke.

IDEAL WEIGHT-LOSS PROGRAM COMPONENTS

Here are some of the qualities of an ideal weight-loss program.
- It's a program that you can and will participate in
- It's a program that has a long-term vision and that incorporates a beginning phase of rapid weight loss, a transition phase of more moderate weight loss, and a long-term maintenance phase
- It's a program that constantly provides new goals to achieve
- It's a program that is clear and unambiguous
- It's a program that delivers results and that has a track record of delivering results

These are the features of the iMetabolic weight-loss program and similar high-quality evidence-based programs around the world. Such programs personalize aspects of their plans that become central to the individual's journey. The program centers offer personal meetings with weight-loss and life coaches, dietary counselors, and psychologists who are specialists in eating behavior and weight loss. iMetabolic and comparable centers have a record of accomplishment via effective, easy-to-follow, successful elements that are central to a successful weight-loss program. The proven use of meal-replacement shakes, effective transition programs, and some very effective long-term maintenance and goal-setting aspects create an atmosphere of success.

A good laugh and a long sleep are the best cures in the doctor's book.

~ Irish proverb

Most likely, if you start a medically supervised weight-loss program at the center you've chosen to attend, you will first be introduced to the staff. Once the staff physician assigned to your case has cleared you to go forward with your weight-loss plan, you'll meet with physical activity specialists who will work with you to put together an exercise program that you can live with. This program will help you incorporate physical activity into your life, hopefully with activities you actually enjoy.

Once the workout plans are in order and you've started getting physical, you'll also start meeting with health and nutrition coaches, psychologists, and behavioral specialists with expertise in the areas of weight and food.

Medically supervised programs vary greatly. Some centers focus on very low-calorie diets: strict diets that allow participants to reduce calories to as little as 600 per day while under direct medical supervision. Others emphasize low-calorie diets, which greatly reduce calories but not so far that direct medical supervision is necessary. Still other centers focus more on particular elements of a weight-loss plan, such as a low-carbohydrate diet, exercise, or group support.

Some programs have proven more effective than others. Most centers don't make the effort to employ *all* the techniques and ideas that have shown success in the past. For example, the vast majority of the commercially available weight-loss centers do not include any type of exercise as part of their plans, even though exercise has been proven to be one of the most important aspects in the battle to lose weight for good. While diet without exercise may result in short-term weight loss, it's not sustainable weight loss. If you don't work out as you lose weight, you will lose lean body mass. The less lean body mass you have, the harder it is to lose weight and the easier it is to put the pounds back on. It's a sure setup for rebound weight gain.

When you're looking for a medically supervised weight-loss program, try to find one that tracks outcomes of all of its patients. Just because one patient lost a stunning amount of weight and kept it off, that doesn't mean that everyone who enrolls in the program will have the same results–that patient's results may have been atypical. A number of medically supervised programs don't collect or report data on patient outcomes, which makes it hard to track successes or even typical results. They're not in business to research weight loss; they're just in business.

But there are doctors, scientists, and centers that *are* studying long-term weight loss.

If you're starting down the road to weight loss, you probably want to know everything you can. Many studies on weight loss have been published in scientific literature, and a few of those studies have made an effort to apply some sophisticated statistical techniques to pool results and data from many studies in many locations.

James Anderson and his colleagues collected data from a large number of published American studies of weight-loss programs and found 29 U.S.-based studies that met the criteria for inclusion in Anderson's own study, which was published in the *American Journal of Clinical Nutrition* in 2001.

An analysis of those 29 studies showed that certain characteristics of weight loss programs lead to higher rates of success; specifically, medically supervised diets of around 800 calories per day appeared to be helpful in terms of achieving long-term weight loss. In fact, weight-loss from these low-calorie diets was significantly greater than weight loss achieved via other types of diets.

Right Doctor, Right Program

The advice in this book comes from an extensive review of the scientific literature and from my own practice and my own experience of helping thousands of patients lose weight successfully and keep it off. The program and methods I describe are all successfully employed by the best medically based weight-loss programs because they work with real people, not just in a lab or a textbook.

Finding and working with the right doctor is a key component of a successful weight-loss program. For many people, this can be the primary care doctor they're already seeing for day-to-day health concerns. Most primary care doctors I know are excellent physicians who do a great job of managing many complex illnesses as well as handling preventative care for their patients. Many have a great deal of knowledge about weight-loss programs and principles, even if the field of medical weight loss isn't the primary focus of their practice. Depending on your own personal situation, you may want to work with your primary care physician if that doctor is well versed in the principles and problems faced during weight gain and obesity, or you may want to find a physician who is experienced at monitoring patients who are participating in vigorous weight-loss programs. If your primary care physician is a good choice, you won't have to spend time finding a different doctor to work with—and you can start your program that much sooner.

If you have serious medical considerations, such as significant heart disease or kidney disease, or you are taking a multitude of medications, then you'll need more active participation and guidance from your physician. Which is fine—most doctors today will applaud your efforts to lose weight, and many have probably encouraged it for years. One more benefit to working with your own primary care physician is your doctor's familiarity with your health concerns and the medications you're taking.

If you don't already have a doctor or if you would be more comfortable working with a specialist, one resource you may want to use is the American Society of Bariatric Physicians (ASBP). The organization's Web site (www.asbp.org) has a physician locator program that can help you find a doctor to work with. A few things that a specialist can do for you from the beginning are:

- Check your body .composition (percentages of fat and muscle in your body) at the start of your weight-loss journey and at various stages of your program
- Check and help you interpret laboratory test results (for cholesterol, kidney function, electrolytes, and other such factors)
- Examine an electrocardiogram of your heart and determine if you have a rare condition known as a prolonged QT interval, which can put you at risk of arrhythmias
- Counsel you about undiagnosed problems related to excessive weight, such as sleep apnea, that might be causing fatigue or headaches

PROGRAMS WITHOUT DOCTORS

You can certainly make the choice to go forward without a doctor. In fact, if it's a choice between going forward on your own and not going forward at all, I applaud your efforts to do it on your own. Certainly, for the overwhelming majority of people in the country, not losing weight is far riskier than losing weight. You may decide you want to proceed on your own after a checkup or you might skip the checkup and just start, figuring you know your body well enough to detect any changes. Almost everyone has dieted at some point, and done it without supervision and without significant adverse effects, so common sense indicates that problems are rare. And it is thoroughly demonstrated that losing lots of unneeded pounds is far safer than continuing to carry those pounds around.

Formally speaking, I recommend that nothing in this book take the place of your own doctor's medical advice. The fact that I'm a physician specializing in weight loss means I've gained valuable experience over the years regarding what works and what doesn't work in terms of achieving healthy weight loss. A specialist can give you tools to work with and help you guard against complications, but your own physician is most familiar with your current health, health concerns, and medications.

Here are some basic recommendations when starting a vigorous medically based weight-loss program:

1. Get a medical checkup and let your doctor know you're embarking on this plan.

2. Consider regular follow-up visits and lab work to check your electrolytes every four to six weeks during the period you're on the shakes-only Induction plan.

3. If you have serious medical conditions, take several medications, or are 55 years old or more, even closer medical monitoring may be warranted.

4. Share your successes: let your doctor know when you've hit some milestones—maybe he or she wants to help other patients in the practice lose weight as well!

If you prefer to work on your own instead of participating in a program through a weight-loss center, I encourage you to meet with your own doctor prior to beginning your program. Your doctor can run a variety of tests that will help you decide what kind and what intensity of program is right for you. These are a few things to discuss:

- Thyroid test

- Periodic routine blood tests of potassium and electrolytes if doing an intense diet

- Tests for problems caused by obesity, such as diabetes, high blood pressure, heart disease, and sleep apnea

- More screening if you're over 50–treadmill test; colonoscopy; mammogram

- Your prescription medications

- Advice about fitness and diet in the context of your personal medical history

SUPPORT AND SABOTAGE

I've said this before, but it bears repeating: You don't have to do this alone. Losing weight is not a one-person challenge–not if you don't want it to be. There are lots of reasons to bring others in on your plans, and probably quite a few reasons to go it alone if you have to.

Friends and family are the people who are going to feel the effects of your weight-loss efforts the most. They're going to be aware of what you're doing even if you've never made a formal declaration of your decision to lose weight. They're going to notice you're eating differently and that you're taking time out of your day to take a walk, go swimming, or go do whatever activity or activities you've decided to take up as your exercise. And they're going to notice when you start losing weight.

Communicate your intentions to your friends and family. Let them in on what you're doing and ask for their support and understanding. At the same time, offer them your own support and understanding, because some of them are going to be confused and unnerved by your changes.

Not everyone will react that way. Some of your friends and family will be enthusiastic for you. They'll offer moral support and celebrations as you hit milestones. They'll shore up your confidence and your determination when the going gets tough. They'll be there for you every step of the way.

Friends are angels who lift us to our feet when our wings have trouble remembering how to fly.

~ Anonymous

COMPLICATIONS

In medicine, we always consider the risks to the patient as well as the benefits when considering any approach in treatment. At this point, I believe the benefits of losing weight have been pretty thoroughly discussed. But because some medically supervised weight-loss programs employ a very low-calorie diet for the first phase of weight loss, I want to look for a moment at the risks to embarking on such a course of treatment.

Comparing risks and benefits of following a medically supervised weight-loss program versus the risks of remaining overweight or obese, it's clear that the risks of remaining overweight are almost always greater than the risks of complications due to following a very low-calorie diet. These complications are rare and shouldn't deter you from working hard at your very low-calorie diet, if that's the course you've chosen for your weight loss, but complications do occur. (See Appendix G for an interview with Dr. Michael J. Bloch for more on risks.)

Diet Risks
Dehydration
If you don't drink enough water, you could become dehydrated or even be at risk for kidney stones. These problems can be avoided simply by drinking adequate fluids and avoiding caffeine (which is a diuretic). You need to consume at least 64 ounces of water daily–that's the eight 8-ounce glasses you've been told about since childhood.

Electrolyte Abnormalities and Low Potassium
Electrolyte abnormalities and low potassium have been reported as side effects of very low-calorie diets and are a good reason to see your doctor and have blood drawn and electrolytes checked during the course of the diet.

Feeling Lightheaded, Fatigued, or Woozy
A radical change in diet, even if it's for the better, can induce a bit of dizziness. Some people have reported headaches several days or weeks into

a very low-calorie diet. It's important to maintain good fluid intake, get plenty of exercise, and maintain adequate consumption of calories and protein, but. you don't want to go back to eating Big Macs if you experience a few headaches or some lightheadedness after you've started a diet. These are symptoms to report to your doctor, but they are usually symptoms that can be worked through.

Protein Deficiency

Protein deficiency is one of the most serious adverse effects of a very low-calorie diet, and it can occur if the diet hasn't been structured properly. A very low-calorie diet that includes fewer than 40 grams of protein per day puts the dieter at risk of wasting too much lean body mass. This can make you feel weaker and more tired. It can also cause you to lose more muscle mass rather than fat mass so that when the diet ends, you're more apt to regain weight than people who had adequate protein intake.

Heart Arrhythmias or Other Serious Problems

A few people may be predisposed to some more serious problems or complications. There is an abnormality of cardiac conduction that can be detected on an EKG; it's known as a prolonged QT interval. Studies have shown that people with this condition may be at elevated risk for arrhythmias while undergoing a very low-calorie diet. This risk is probably quite small, but it's important to have it identified by a physician.

Other Risks

A medically based weight-loss program that involves marked reduction in carbohydrate intake may cause constipation as a side effect. In addition, some people find they don't tolerate certain kinds of meal replacements particularly well, and they may have indigestion, nausea, headaches, or other side effects (usually a change to a different brand or different flavor of shake can solve this problem). There are also psychological side effects in adhering to a challenging weight-loss program. which can add stress to people's lives.

116

Gallstones are a risk, as well. There's still uncertainty in the medical community as to whether losing weight brings out gallstones, which would have become symptomatic later in life anyway, or whether the metabolic changes lead to the formation of symptomatic gallstones. Either way, there's about an X-percent increase in the incidence of gallstone troubles with significant weight loss. (Keep in mind that the main risk factors for gallstone disease are being overweight or obese, being female and having the associated female hormones circulating in the bloodstream, age, childbirth, and pregnancies. Yes, this means that gallstones are more common in women than in men, but it's a very common condition among all people, young or old, overweight or normal weight.)

At our center, we've also heard complaints of nausea, vomiting, diarrhea, and rashes. All of these kinds of symptoms can be experienced by people whether or not they're following a weight-loss program but, since we're paying closer attention to people in our center and our clinic, we're aware of these symptoms more than we would be otherwise.

The adverse effects noted are as follows: constipation (68 percent of the low-carbohydrate group reported experiencing this, versus 35 percent of the low-fat group); headache (60 percent versus 40 percent); halitosis (38 percent versus 8 percent); muscle cramps (35 percent versus 7 percent); diarrhea (23 percent versus 7 percent); general weakness (25 percent versus 8 percent); and rash (13 percent versus 0 percent).

To date, studies on medically supervised weight-loss programs have not indicated a risk of severe or catastrophic problems such as heart attacks, fatal arrhythmias, suicide, stroke, seizures, or other major events.

Exercise Risks

The weight-loss program that you are going to enroll in will have an exercise component. As I mentioned, the importance of this exercise program cannot be over-emphasized. Nonetheless, some people are not healthy enough for strenuous exercise. It's important for your health to be evaluated to determine if you should have a cardiac stress test or other evaluations prior to enrolling in any vigorous new physical activity.

Sometimes people want to start a completely new life, and do it with enthusiasm, all at once. They very enthusiastically start in on a low-calorie diet and they want to hit the gym right away–and hit it hard. For some of these folks who haven't been exercising regularly for many years and who have become seriously overweight, a gentler initiation that includes regular walking would be a better way to start–after a cardiac stress test. These folks might benefit from lipid-lowering drugs and other interventions to reduce their cardiac risk in addition to the weight loss program.

If you're enrolling in an official program with a weight-loss center, it's still a good idea to check in with your own physician, who has an entire file on your overall health and who will be able to point out areas where you should take extra care or even point out benefits you haven't expected. It's an extra step, but it's worth it for your health–and you can schedule it right now as you get started on your weight-loss program.

Risks must be taken, because the greatest hazard in life is to risk nothing.

~ Leo Buscaglia

6

.
.
.

Phase One: Induction

When someone comes into our center to embark upon a weight-loss journey, we work with that individual to put together a weight-loss plan that includes a goal of losing at least 30 to 40 pounds in 90 days. We refer to this as the Induction phase. The first thing we do is figure out a calorie deficit that will produce the kind of weight loss desired.

If you take the baseline figure of approximately 2,500 calories a day to sustain normal daily activity, and subtract 500 calories from that daily total, you'll be looking at a weight loss of approximately 12 pounds at the end of the three months. Most of the time, we're looking for a bigger loss than that. A 1,500-calorie-a-day deficit moves the person closer to a weight loss of 40 pounds during that time. To create a calorie deficit of 1,500 calories daily, take 1,500 from the baseline, 2,500, and you're left with 1,000 calories. This is not atypical of many diet plans. The "1,000 calories a day" mark is the essential low-calorie diet.

At iMetabolic, we evaluate the patient and determine if an even more rigorous diet is called for. If so, we will move to a net intake of 850 calories daily for phase one–Induction. The difference in daily caloric intake isn't really that great, but 850 calories will result in a slightly greater number of pounds lost. The 1,000-calorie diet is very similar, but it allows for some leeway in terms of the inclusion of vegetables and some other food options. It's a little easier to follow–or swallow–for three months.

The decision to follow an 850-calorie plan or a 1,000-calorie plan is based partly on the person's desire for weight loss and partly on health issues. Someone with serious health conditions might be better off with 1,000 calories a day. Everyone could probably stick with 1,000 calories daily with little in the way of health troubles or significant side effects. But I always recommend you get the advice of your doctor.

While the best results come from committing to this program for 90 days, some people find this simply too long a period to go without "real food"; others stay on it for 180 days or even longer. But try to agree to commit to it for a period of 90 days, and if you can do more before making a Transition, then you're off to a magnificent start on your weight-loss journey.

THE FIRST 90 DAYS

For your 90-day Induction phase, I suggest you follow a liquid protein meal-replacement program, possibly with protein bars in addition to meal-replacement shakes. There are a couple of reasons this works. First, it eliminates the problem of choice. You don't need to worry about what you're going to eat for your next meal (and what you might possibly cheat with just a little bit during your next meal) because your next meal is exactly the same as your last meal: a protein shake.

In addition, there are a good many protein powders you can mix up yourself and pre-mixed low-sugar, high-protein shakes you can buy that contain 150 to 260 calories per shake. Right there you've made things easier by being able to track your calories at a glance and keep your carbohydrates low and your protein high. If each shake is 150 calories, you can have four shakes throughout the day and be at 600 calories, which equals 800 calories—what do you eat to get the remaining 50 calories (if you're on the 850-calorie plan)? What about if you're on the 1,000-calorie plan?

The second benefit of following a liquid protein meal-replacement program is that it's a chance to get away from the bad foods in your diet right away. The fast foods, the snack foods, and the high-calorie, high-fat, and high-carbohydrate foods are gone right away, and there's no way to cheat—each meal is just a protein shake or bar.

The protein component is important—you want to maintain lean body mass and burn fat, so you need to get at least 100 grams of protein a day to promote maintenance of lean body mass during this rapid weight loss. If you're in good health with no existing kidney concerns, even eating as much as 120 grams of protein a day will be fine. You can drop to as low as 60 grams if you find it difficult to get that much protein into your diet, although, at that level, you risk burning lean muscle mass instead of fat.

The only concern with a high intake of protein (around 120 grams a day) comes into play if you have any kind of kidney damage or renal insufficiency. Kidney function problems can make it easier for kidneys to become overloaded and lose the ability to process all that protein. High intake of proteins can also cause a rise in serum protein byproducts and make kidney dysfunction worse. But such cases are rare, and they are usually easily detected with a routine blood test.

Some centers only offer one kind of meal replacement, in part because it is profitable for them. Although we at iMetabolic designed and created a specific line of meal-replacement shakes based on our patients' comments, tastes, and weight loss experience, our center offers a range of meal-replacement protein powders and shakes from various companies. The only real requirement in finding a protein powder that works for you is to find high-quality medical-grade protein powders with sufficient protein and a good combination of vitamins and amino acids (the building blocks of protein and lean body mass). Read the labels and make sure that the protein content is high and that the carb content is low.

Spend a little time comparison shopping for your protein meal replacement. They're not the cheapest things in the world, and really, you don't want to purchase the cheapest protein meal replacement available anyway. You're going to be eating very little else for the next 90 days. In fact, whether or not protein bars are included in your meal plan, you're going to be relying almost exclusively on liquid protein meal-replacement shakes for the next three months.

You can find protein meal replacements, even high quality ones, in some interesting places. Aside from your grocery store and specialty stores such as nutrition and vitamin stores, you can find good brands with high protein and low carbs in places like Costco and through the Internet retailer Amazon (www.amazon.com).

The very simplicity of following a meal-replacement program makes it doable. I've worked personally with a great many people who have followed this program, and they've all gotten through it.

To succeed, we must first believe that we can.

~ Michael Korda

I am so grateful that I found the iMetabolic program. I had struggled with ever-increasing weight for a number of years. I made half-hearted attempts at dieting on my own but just couldn't seem to stay with anything. The structure of the program made it almost easy to adhere to. I live alone, and I tended to snack a lot or eat the wrong things rather than prepare food for myself. Having the protein meal replacements at the prescribed six times was an easy way for me to eat regularly and get much better nutrition. I had plenty of energy, which surprised me, and I really didn't feel hungry.

It was so great to watch the weight finally come off every week! I no longer have to shop in the "fat girl" stores. I feel so much better about how I look! I had hip surgery a year ago, and I know that the weight loss made a difference in my recovery time and in the long-term outcome of the surgery. Thank you, iMetabolic!

Tamara Moyer–lost 39.5 pounds

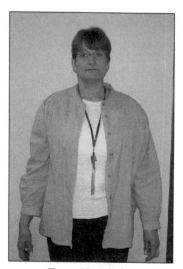

Tamara Moyer (Before)

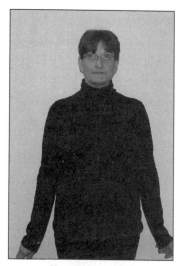

Tamara Moyer (After)

BEGINNING INDUCTION

The first few days of the program might make 90 days feel impossible. But before you start to think you're not going to get through this or you can't make it 90 days without a cheeseburger or cheesecake, there are a few facts for you to take into account.

First off, not only have tens of thousands of people gone before you in programs like this one and lived to tell the tale but, in addition, these decreases and the program doesn't seem that difficult after all. This makes complete sense, given the biology.

There's a biochemical reaction taking place at the beginning of the program when you've made such a big jump from normal calories (probably too many calories) to a low-calorie diet. In the beginning of the program, people go into a mild state of ketosis as the body's store of adipose tissue—fat—is broken down by the liver. These byproducts include fatty acids, which are burned to make energy, and ketones (waste products left after fat is converted to energy), which are washed through the bloodstream. This is the beginning of weight loss. (It's actually best to be in only a mild state of ketosis, otherwise, the body becomes alarmed that you're burning too many energy stores, slows the metabolism way down, and refuses to burn any extra calories it already has or can get hold of.)

You'll probably also find that your appetite has decreased after the second or third day. Once appetite decreases, most people find the diet fairly easy to stay on for the entire three months. I've guided many, many people through this diet, and the majority of them reported not only that they experienced a decrease in appetite during the first week, but also that motivation was enough to drive them. If they were hungry during the first few days, they took it in stride.

Motivation

There's no question about it: if your motivation isn't in place, it's going to be pretty darned hard to stay on this plan for the full 90 days–which is why, before you embark on your 3-month journey, you're going to sit down, map out your goals, and put down in writing what you want to accomplish, how much weight you're going to lose, how much weight will be left to lose after the 90 days is over, how wonderful you're going to feel when you've lost the weight, and how you're going to have more energy and confidence and just be happier all the way around.

Take a moment to write down your 90-day goals, including the weight-loss figures that represent personal milestones. Your list may look something like this:

My 90 Days
Current weight: _____
Goal weight: _____
Goal weight at day 90: _____
Type of exercise: _____
Milestone weight at day 180: _____
Milestone weight at day 360: _____

Maintenance weight: _____

Celebrations: _____

My motivation: Why I'm powering up to lose 40 pounds in 90 days: _____

KEEP ON TRACK

If the going does get tough, that's the time to go back and review your goals. Before you're tempted to cheat, before you fall off the liquid protein meal-replacement wagon, remind yourself of the activities you want to pursue once you lose the weight. Are there trips you plan to take or specific clothes you want to buy? Is there an event coming up that you want to trim down for, or do you want to rid yourself of some troublesome medical conditions? Whatever your goals, they're worth it. Don't let something as small as 90 days–three months–one quarter of a year–stand in the way of achieving your dreams.

> *If you don't do what's best for your body, you're the one who comes up on the short end.*
>
> ~ Julius Erving

Keep in mind, as well, that you will start transitioning out of the Induction phase around week eight of your 90 days. So, while it is important to be strict and vigilant as long as you can, your range of options does widen before the 90 days is out.

So Much So Soon

If you've been overweight and struggling to lose weight for a long time, there are many advantages to losing so much weight so quickly. For one thing, losing 40 pounds in just three months gives you a tremendous feeling of confidence and accomplishment. You'll have a new appreciation for what you can do and you'll not only be jump-starting your weight loss, but your confidence and drive as well.

For another, if you're carrying 40 or more pounds of excess weight, your health is suffering as a result. If you have at least 40 pounds to lose, you're already putting a strain on your body and you may already be dealing with basic health challenges.

An individual who has a BMI of 25 or more is considered overweight. Every five pounds of body weight raises the BMI another unit (roughly) and every additional unit of BMI increases the risk of health complications.

Here's the good news: the instant you start losing the weight, your risk of health complications drops. People who lose 20 or 30 pounds find their blood pressure dropping and their cholesterol numbers coming into line, and they find themselves in a healthier place altogether. Every pound lost lowers the risk of health complications and increases good health. Every pound. Even a little goes a long way.

But, for some people, weight loss simply isn't about health. Although I'm not promoting weight loss for cosmetic reasons, if wanting to look better motivates you to lose weight, there's nothing wrong with that! I had one patient who wanted to lose weight for a reunion. While I emphasized all the health-related reasons for him to lose weight, he went on thinking about looking good at his reunion–which was fine, because it gave him motivation and he lost the weight, and the health benefits came right along with the weight loss, even though the health benefits weren't at the top of his concerns. My job in a case like that is to help my patient reach the goals set and to explain the long-term benefits of the weight loss. Then we look for another event to help him keep the weight off the next year and the year after that.

*My weight is always perfect for my height—
which varies.*

~ Nicole Hollander

90-DAY LIQUID DIET

Boiled down to a few essential principles, here's a powerful diet plan for initial weight loss.

For the Induction phase, I recommend a diet that contains 850 to 1,000 calories per day.

Key Principles

- Commit to success. This is a temporary Induction program. You can do it.
- During this 90-day period, you will not be consuming any other foods or beverages than those included in these guidelines.
- Use eight scoops of iMetabolic meal-replacement shake mix (or equivalent) every day. Using the prescribed amount will help ensure that you are getting all the nutrients you need.
- Eat at regularly scheduled times. You will need to eat five to six times per day, allowing not more than two to three hours between eating intervals.
- Mix your powdered shake mix with water only. It will blend best if you use a blender, but it's fine if mixed in a shaker cup.
- Adding any fruit or other ingredients to your shake means accounting for those added calories. It is OK to add sugar-free flavorings, such as cooking extracts, sugar-free flavored syrups, sugar-free JELL-O® powder, or Crystal Light® powder.
- Consume 64 fluid ounces of calorie-free liquid each day in addition to your shakes. These liquids may include:

- Water
- Crystal Light®
- Propel® enhanced water
- Fruit2O® enhanced water
- Sugar-free Kool-Aid®
- Iced tea (unsweetened or sweetened with sugar substitute only)
- Coffee (unsweetened or sweetened with sugar substitute only)
- Fat-free broth

If you're hungry, you may have the following

- Vegetables, raw or cooked. Limit your portion to two cups daily. Do not add any oils, sauces, butter, salad dressings, or other condiments that contain calories. You may add flavored vinegars, lemon juice, salt, or spices.
- Asparagus
- Broccoli
- Cauliflower
- Celery
- Cucumbers
- Crookneck or zucchini squash
- Green, red, yellow, or orange sweet peppers
- Lettuce (up to FOUR cups daily)
- Mushrooms
- Onion
- Radishes
- Spinach

Calorie/Protein Content for the Induction Phase

Meal/Snack	Food/Supplement*	Approximate Calories	Approximate Protein
Breakfast:	2 scoops protein shake mix plus water	180 calories	26 grams
Morning snack:	Protein bar	150–160 calories	15 grams
Lunch:	2 scoops protein shake mix plus water	180 calories	26 grams
Afternoon snack:	1 scoop protein shake mix plus water	90 calories	15 grams
Dinner:	1 scoop protein shake mix plus water; selected vegetable	250 calories	26 grams
Evening snack:	1 scoop protein shake mix plus water	90 calories	15grams

Total calories: 950–960
Total grams of protein: 125 (approximate)

A 90-calorie protein shake may be substituted for the protein bar, resulting in a saving of approximately 40 to 70 calories per day.

Two items of fruit may be added to this diet, with an estimated 200 calories added.

iMetabolic Supplements	Approximate Calories	Approximate Proteins	Approximate Carbohydrate	Approximate Fat
Puddings	80 calories	12 grams	5–11 grams	0–0.5 grams
Hot beverages	70 calories	12 grams	5–6 grams	0.5–1 grams
Shakes	90 calories	12 grams	9–11 grams	0–0.5 grams
Fruit drinks	60 calories	12 grams	2–3 grams	0 grams
Soups	70 calories	12 grams	5–7 grams	0 grams
Per supplement	80 calories	12 grams	5–8 grams	0.5 grams

Following this protocol, you will remain within your target range of 800 to 1,000 calories per day and ensure an aggressive, but safe, weight loss.

This diet may seem boring–and it is. It's *simple*, and that's why it works. We'll introduce some excitement into your diet after you lose weight.

It must be emphasized that if any of these programs (which have been developed through years of research and trials) are to work, they must be followed to the letter. Any variations on your part will lead to less weight loss. This is not a program in which you have a great deal of food choices. Stick with it for 90 days and you will see amazing results.

AVOIDING SABOTAGE

One of the points of the liquid protein meal-replacement program is that, after the first couple of days on the program, you're not going to be hungry. The fact that you're not suffering from hunger pangs makes it easier not to cheat or fall off the wagon and eat something you're not supposed to, but you're probably well aware that there are all kinds of ways to mess up on a diet without meaning to.

If you work around other people, food is going to be available, and this will certainly be an issue. Workplaces always seem to have somebody who wants to cook for everyone or bring in baked goods. There's often a candy dish or an open box of cookies (left, quite possibly, by someone who only wanted a few pieces, then left the rest to tempt everyone else). Then there are working lunches, drinks after work, and myriad birthdays to celebrate. Even if your work consists of doing something physical outdoors, chances are that you are exposed to vending machines, candy dishes, boxes of doughnuts, "roach coaches," and that obnoxious (but well-intentioned!) person who loves to bake.

You're going to have to ignore it all. Just put your blinders on and act as if none of it is there. Think up something to tell coworkers when they're actually standing in your office doorway offering food and you don't take it.

And keep drinking your shakes and eating your bars. If you work a regular eight-hour day (or night), make sure you're eating at fairly regularly spaced intervals. If you skip a shake with the misguided intention to lose weight more quickly, you're apt to get too hungry and end up with significantly lowered willpower—which can result in eating something you shouldn't. Plus, you put your metabolic engine at risk by putting the supply chain at risk and, therefore, telling the metabolism to "slow down and store more". Remember, this is the exact opposite of what we are trying to do here.

If you're pushed for time, look for pre-mixed protein shakes in individual servings. They cost a bit more and they're not environmentally friendly with all that extra packaging, but you're not going to be doing this forever, and it's important.

In between your shakes, and before you're confronted with an office meeting where there's going to be food or during the long afternoon before you go home, when hunger sneaks up, have a protein bar. Look for one that has, preferably, fewer than 200 calories, fewer than 10 grams of carbohydrates, and a high percentage of protein. One of the few nice things to come out of the obesity epidemic is the range of different products available. I suggest you stay with a protein bar, some of which taste more like cookies and treats than something healthy, but if you have a better chance of success if there's something crunchy or salty or both in your afternoon, then check out the low-calorie, low-carb, crunchy snacks available to you. Optimally, you're looking for something that contains 150 to 170 calories and at least 15 grams of protein.

Most protein powders and pre-mixed shakes come in vanilla, chocolate, and strawberry flavors. If you're having three shakes a day for 90 days, that's 90 servings of each flavor. That can get pretty dull and hard to swallow pretty quickly.

Look for low-carb, high-quality protein powders in a variety of flavors (such as orange and banana) so you won't get bored.

And, if that isn't enough, pick up a copy of *Shakin' It Up!*, a great book by Chef Dave Fouts (it's available on the iMetabolic Web site at www.imetabolic.com/store/weight-loss-books-c-9.html). It offers a variety of recipes you can make using extracts and flavorings that add negligible calories but change up the taste of what you're drinking.

The rest of the three months is very close to what you've already been doing. You're building on your momentum. You've already lost weight, which feels *great,* and now you're building your enthusiasm for the remainder of the 12 weeks.

INDUCTION AND EXERCISE

You need to use your muscles consistently throughout your rapid weight loss so that you send biochemical and hormonal signals through your body that lean body mass needs to be utilized and sustained. So, instead of breaking down your muscles and cannibalizing them for nutrients, you're continuing to develop protein stores in the bloodstream and taking in sufficient amounts of vitamins and cofactors (minerals and other molecules that assist the cell machinery in protein synthesis) to build muscle mass and sustain it through weight loss.

We will either find a way or make one.

~ Hannibal

If you haven't been exercising, start slowly. Taking a nice, brisk walk is a perfect way to incorporate exercise into your day. You can do it before work, on breaks, at lunch, or after work–or all of the above, if your legs feel ready for it. Find a pedometer (they're sold by many different retailers, including Walmart, running stores, the online retailer Amazon, and the online products store at iMetabolic's Web site). Work up to the goal of something like 10,000 steps a day (roughly equivalent to five miles–500 calories out of the equation). The nice thing is, those steps don't have to be taken all at once. Park farther away from your office. Take a walk at lunch. Take another after dinner. Watch your steps add up while you realize you're doing something wonderful for yourself. (For more information on walking, see Chapter 9 and Appendix D.)

Life itself is the proper binge.

~ Julia Child

Two of my clients who had been swimmers earlier in their lives were encouraged to take up swimming as their form of exercise, and they took to it readily, finding a new zest for physical activity that had been missing in their lives. Once in the water, the joint and back pain associated with standing and walking on dry land was gone. While swimming wasn't easy, it was easier than walking. Both patients found exercise programs and an indoor pool that held swimming classes that catered to their age groups, so they were able to exercise regularly, improve their health, and make some new friends.

For a third client, even swimming proved too difficult, but he was able to use small hand weights, and he started getting regular exercise while sitting and watching his favorite programs on the History Channel. He simply agreed he wouldn't watch television unless his arms were busy with those weights. He took this as a challenge and did so religiously, imaging that his arms were the battery that was powering the television.

Sometimes it takes a little creativity, but there are ways to get regular exercise for everybody.

A Little Disclaimer

Will everyone lose 40 pounds in 90 days? Of course not. Someone starting this program with 40 pounds to lose may find that, as the program continues and the goal weight gets closer, the weight loss slows down. At the beginning of a weight-loss program, it's easier to lose weight because there's more weight to lose. Someone who needs to lose 200 pounds will probably lose more weight more quickly at the beginning than someone with less weight to lose because there is more weight to be lost. Over the course of the 90 days, the person with more to lose may lose a great deal more than 40 pounds. As the program progresses, there's less weight to lose, so weight loss slows. So, at the end of your 90 days, if you only had 40 pounds to lose in the first place, you may have lost it all—or you may still have a small amount of weight to lose. I use 40 pounds as an example because it is a challenging, yet achievable, goal if you follow the directions and don't cheat. If you've lost it all, you'll move into Maintenance. If there's more to lose, you might want to stay with the Induction phase a bit longer.

The amount of weight you can lose in the 90-day Induction phase varies from person to person. It certainly varies depending on the degree to which people stick to the program and don't cheat. Someone who sticks religiously to the program and complies rigorously with the diet and exercise components will lose more weight and burn more calories than someone who doesn't. It's common sense.

If you're interested in getting a feel for what a medically based weight-loss center looks and feels like or you want to learn about tools available to you online, visit www.imetabolic.com.

---

90 Days Is Just the Beginning

Forty pounds is a great achievement, but it is really just the beginning. Induction, whether it results in 20 or 80 pounds lost, and whether it lasted 60 days or 180, is meant to be the kick-starter of a longer program. Even though you've lost the weight in a healthy way and preserved lean body mass, you're still at risk for gradual weight gain if you don't pay attention to the components involved in long-term weight loss and weight maintenance.

You need to be aware of the risk of rebound weight gain and of plateaus you can hit as you continue your weight-loss program. You need to remember how important nutrition is and not allow yourself to gain and lose weight over and over. There aren't any shortcuts. The "40 pounds in 90 days" approach is a relatively short-term strategy for healthy weight loss, but I want to emphasize that it's meant to be viewed as the beginning of changes that will last a lifetime.

7

. . .

Phase Two: Transition

At the end of the 90 days, you will have lost 40 or more pounds and either achieved your weight-loss goals or made huge strides forward in that direction. Congratulations! If you've followed all the steps and continued with the program as it's laid out, you've not only lost the weight, but you've also developed a few new behaviors. You've learned to set goals, changed how you interact with friends and family, figured out what you do when confronted with foods you weren't planning on eating, learned how to say no to calories you don't want—no matter how well-intentioned the person offering them is—identified some of your triggers, and begun to make exercise part of your daily life. You've lost anywhere from two to four or more pounds every week, and you're looking forward to some of the activities you've been planning or to some new clothes, a vacation, or a special event.

This is all important. It's important to keep the short-term goals in sight, and I hope you've kept your promises to yourself and rewarded your good behaviors and celebrated those weight-loss milestones.

It's equally important to keep the long-term considerations in mind. This is the time to transition from your short-term eating and exercising behaviors to the long-term behaviors you're going to institute in order to keep the weight off permanently. This is where the challenge lies. You've probably experienced rebound weight gain at some point in your life, and now's not the time to experience it again. So, starting in week eight of your 90-day Induction phase, you're going to begin to move into the Transition phase. This involves introducing real foods into the mix and learning about portion sizes. If you've been very successful in your weight loss, you might start having a carefully designed meal for dinner in week 10.

One way to make certain you don't go overboard is to eat meals with carefully controlled portions. You can certainly prepare your own meals, with an eye toward carb, fat, and protein content, or you can obtain prepared meals from centers and kitchens that focus on healthy meals and dietary restrictions (search online for shelf-stable prepared meals and compare them to those from our center).

Whichever route you choose, it's important to understand that each meal is not going to top out much past 300 or maybe 350 calories. Even though that's a relatively low calorie count, it's still higher than the protein shakes you've been having, so you're losing some of your calorie deficit. It's a small shift, but it's a good time to increase the exercise you've been doing to avoid losing all of the benefits of the calorie deficit you've already created.

Begin to work the meals into your days while you continue with exercise and daily shakes. Focus now on the rest of your weight-loss journey, whether you have more weight to lose or you are ready to move to the Maintenance phase. This is the time to look at behavioral techniques, to continue reading labels, to look for different forms of exercise you enjoy, and to further take advantage of all the other tips and tools you've learned along the way so far.

When the 90 days is up, you're not going to revert back to your old eating habits. You're going to be staying at a fairly low calorie count. I suggest you continue to make visits to your weight-loss center or to your physician so that you can continue to track your weight loss.

Success leaves clues.

~ Jim Rohn

If you're part of a support group, don't stop attending! Not only is it a good idea to stay in contact with people who are experiencing the same things you are and who can encourage you as you start moving into the world of real food again, but again; in addition, now's the time that you can encourage others who are just starting on their journey. And that feels wonderful.

Studies very clearly show that most people who lose weight will gain it back in the long run *unless* they stick to long-term behavior changes, activities, and eating plans.

Your long-term success at achieving and sustaining weight loss is so important to your health and well-being, it's worth every bit of struggle; every penny you spend, every minute you pursue it. And you *can* do it.

PSYCHOLOGISTS AND NUTRITIONISTS

If you're working through a weight-loss center, there's a good chance that you'll have an appointment or two with the psychologist there. Psychologists who work with weight-loss centers have experience working with people who are making the changes you're making in your life. They're experts in behavior modification and all other aspects of the psychology of the weight-loss journey.

Sitting down with a psychologist before you begin your program can be very valuable. A psychologist can offer insight about what will work for you and offer suggestions and feedback on things that you might think about or work on changing in order to be successful. Few candidates are ever turned away because of psychological evaluations, though some are found to have deeper emotional issues that require some counseling while moving forward.

Seeing a psychologist on such a limited basis and only on the topics of your upcoming weight loss and positive life change doesn't mean you've gone into therapy. But, if you do have concerns about the changes you're making in your life and how others might react to them, many of these professionals are willing to work with you on an ongoing basis.

In the same way, talking to a nutritionist can help you pinpoint changes you need to make in your eating habits and behaviors. A nutritionist can explain the ins and outs of nutrition and help you put together an individualized eating plan for your Transition and Maintenance phases.

If the program you're in offers the opportunity to talk with a psychologist and a nutritionist, I urge you to do so–both professionals can offer great insight and a healthy leg up on your new life. If you're following this program on your own, I urge you to invest in a couple of appointments with both professionals–you can ask your doctor for referrals or recommendations. Any opportunity that helps you succeed and achieve your goals is worthwhile.

TRANSITION DIET

The Transition period lasts as long as it takes you to lose the remainder of the weight you want to drop. I recommend you plan on sticking with this phase for several months (12 to 24 weeks is typical). With the right attitude, commitment, and support, you can do this; you can lose the weight. Moreover, you can avoid rebound weight gain and keep it off!

For the Transition phase, I recommend a diet that contains 1,000 to 1,500 calories per day.

1,000-1,500 calories/day

Key Principles

- Commit to success. This phase takes discipline and commitment. You can do it.
- During the Transition phase, you will need to track closely your calories and carbohydrate intake.
- Continue to rely on protein-based meal-replacement shakes and bars for snacks and some meals.

Phase two, Transition, is designed to allow you the option to make daily choices in food. The advantage of this program is the freedom to choose *real food*. The disadvantage is that you have the freedom to choose any foods–and sometimes you can make the wrong food choices.

This is a good time to master the art of journaling your diet. Weighing foods, measuring foods, counting calories, and counting fat and carbohydrate grams are all necessary if you are to continue your weight loss in this phase of the program.

During the Transition phase, you'll probably experience increased hunger brought on by real foods, so be prepared for it. You don't have to satisfy every hunger pang. Get used to living with it. In time, it becomes less acute. Remember that calories from simple carbohydrates, such as sugar, actually make you hungrier after the blood sugar surge is gone, so try to avoid them.

> When you're in the Transition phase, don't forget to continue eating five to six meals per day while keeping protein as your number one focus. This is a critical long-term strategy that will help keep hunger at bay, help keep your metabolism running well, and fuel your lean-body mass.

Phase two, Transition, features a high-protein, low-fat, low-carb diet. Each morning you begin the day by having some protein, and each evening you end the day with another helping of protein. You begin the morning with a medically formulated protein shake for breakfast. A protein bar is used as a mid-morning snack or, if you are dining out for lunch, is eaten one hour prior to lunch to help suppress your appetite.

For both lunch and dinner, we urge our clients to make a recipe from the Chef Dave cookbook or to choose a prepared meal. Each lunch and dinner should contain between 300 and 500 calories. As a mid-afternoon snack or one hour prior to having dinner, you have another protein bar. The evening snack is either a protein shake or a protein bar.

It's up to you to make the choices and to ramp up the physical activities that will produce additional weight loss in this phase.

The following few tables break down some specifics of the Transition phase of your diet.

Diet Schedule for the Transition Phase

Time	Location	Situation	Food Type
7:00 a.m.	Home kitchen	Breakfast	Protein shake* and vitamin
8:45 a.m.	Work or home	Snack	Coffee or tea
10:30 a.m.	Work or home	Snack	Protein bar
12:15 p.m.	Work or home	Lunch	300- to 400-calorie meal
2:00 p.m.	Work or home	Snack	Water
3:15 p.m.	Work or home	Snack	Protein bar
4:45 p.m.	Work or home	Snack	Coffee or tea
6:15 p.m.	Home kitchen	Dinner	300 to 500-calorie meal
8:00 p.m.	Home	Snack	Diet soda
9:30 p.m.	Home	Snack	Protein bar

Sample 1,200-Calorie Meal Plan for the Transition Phase

Breakfast

Choose ONE (starch)	½ cup cereal (hot or cold) with ½ cup skim milk ½ bagel (1 ounce) or English muffin 1 slice toast: white, whole wheat, or rye 1 reduced-fat or fat-free waffle with 2 tablespoons sugar-free syrup
Choose ONE (fruit)	Fresh: 1 small banana, apple, orange, nectarine, or peach or ¾ cup berries or 1 cup melon or ½ grapefruit Canned: ½ cup fruit in natural juices Juice: ½ cup orange, pineapple, or apple
Choose ONE (milk)	1 cup skim or 1% milk or 1 cup nonfat or low-fat yogurt (plain or fruit flavored with artificial sweetener)
Choose ONE (optional)	1 teaspoon reduced-fat margarine or 2 teaspoons low-sugar jam or jelly 1 tablespoon fat-free cream cheese or 1 tablespoon nondairy creamer
Non-caloric beverages:	6–12 ounces coffee, tea, calorie-free beverage or water
Choose ONE	Daily multivitamin

Mid-morning snack
Choose ONE   Protein shake or bar

NOTE: Water intake should add up to at least 8 cups daily (64 ounces)

Lunch

Choose ONE (starch)

2 slices "diet" (40-calorie) bread:
white, whole wheat, or rye (80 calories)

Choose ONE (meat)

2 ounces skinless chicken or turkey breast,
2 ounces boiled shrimp
2 ounces tuna packed in water
2 ounces fat-free cheese

Choose ONE OR MORE
(vegetables)

2 cups total of lettuce, tomato, carrots,
celery, cabbage, cucumber, mushrooms,
onion, peppers, broccoli, or cauliflower

Choose ONE (fruit)

Fresh: 1 small banana, apple, orange,
nectarine or peach or ¾ cup berries or
1 cup melon or ½ grapefruit
Canned: ½ cup fruit in natural juices

Non-caloric beverages

6 to 12 ounces sugar-free, calorie-free
beverage (such as Crystal Light or
calorie-free soda) or low-sodium
bouillon or water

Mid-afternoon snack

Choose ONE OR MORE
(optional)

Protein shake or bar

NOTE: Water intake should add up to at least 8 cups daily (64 ounces)

Dinner

Choose ONE (starch)	3 ounces baked or boiled potato (about 1/2 potato) ½ pita bread 1 ounce reduced-fat crackers ½ cup pasta, rice, corn, peas, or mashed potato ½ hot dog or hamburger bun 1 ounce piece bread or roll
Choose ONE (meat)	3 ounces baked or broiled lean beef, pork, veal, lamb or salmon 1 reduced-fat hot dog
Choose ONE (vegetable)	1/2 cup raw, steamed, or boiled asparagus, green beans broccoli, carrots, cauliflower, spinach, summer squash, tomato sauce or zucchini 1 cup total raw lettuce, tomato, carrots, celery, cabbage, cucumber, mushrooms, onion, pepper, watercress
Choose ONE (fat)	1 teaspoon butter or margarine 2 teaspoons peanut butter 1 tablespoon regular salad dressing or 2 tablespoons reduced-fat salad dressing

· ·

NOTE: Water intake should add up to at least 8 cups daily (64 ounces)

Dinner *(continued)*

Choose ONE (optional)	1 tablespoon fat-free mayonnaise or salad dressing
	2 teaspoons peanut butter
	1 tablespoon coconut
	1 tablespoon taco sauce
	1/4 cup salsa
Non-caloric beverages	6–12 ounces calorie-free beverage, low-sodium bouillon, or water

Evening snack

Choose ONE	Protein shake or bar

....

NOTE: Water intake should add up to at least 8 cups daily (64 ounces)

1,200-Calorie Meal Plan Nutritional Parameters for the Transition Phase

BREAKFAST	Calories	Protein	Carbohydrates	Fat
One starch	80	3 grams	15 grams	≤1 grams
One fruit	60	–	15 grams	–
One milk	90	8 grams	12 grams	0–3 grams
One optional	10*	–	<5 grams	<0.5 grams
Calorie-free beverage	0	–	–	–
Subtotal	**230–240 calories**	**11 grams**	**42–47 grams**	**0.5–3 grams**
LUNCH				
One starch	80	3 grams	15 grams	≤1 grams
One meat	55–70	7–14 grams	–	0–3 grams
One vegetable	50	4 grams	10 grams	–
One fruit	60	–	15 grams	–
One fat				
One optional	10*	–	<5 grams	<0.5 grams
Calorie-free beverage	0	–	–	–
Sub-total	**290–315 calories**	**14–21 grams**	**40–45 grams**	**5–9 grams**
DINNER				
One starch	80	3 grams	15 grams	≤1 grams
Meat: 4 ounces very lean	140	28 grams	–	0–4 grams
or 3 ounces lean	(165)	(21 grams)	(–)	(9 grams)
2 vegetables	50	4 grams	10 grams	–
One fat	45	–	–	5 grams
One optional	10*	–	<5 grams	<0.5 grams
Non-caloric beverage	0	–	–	–
Sub-total	**315–350 calories**	**28–35 grams**	**25–30 grams**	**5–15 grams**
Total from Meals	**835–905 calories**	**53–67 grams**	**107–122 grams**	**10.5–27 grams**

Target = 890 calories   * Optional (free) food choices are 10 calories on average; typical range = 0–20 calories per serving.

iMetabolic Supplements	Calories	Protein	Carbohydrates	Fat
Protein bars	160	15 grams	7–11 grams	3–5 grams
Gelatin	60	15 grams	0 grams	0 grams
Hot beverages	90	15 grams	4–5 grams	0.5–1.5 grams
Protein shake mix (1 scoop)	90	14 grams	9–11 grams	0–0.5 grams
Fruit drinks	70	15 grams	2–3 grams	0 grams
Soups	80	16 grams	3–4 grams	0 grams
Per supplement	**90**	**15 grams**	**5–8 grams**	**0.5 grams**

Totals:				
2 supplements	180	30 grams	10–16 grams	1 gram

	Calories	Protein	Carbohydrate	Fat
1,200-Calorie Plan	1,145–1,215	87–101 grams	136–159 grams	16.5–33 grams
Percent of calories: Typical range depending on food choices		25–35%	50–55%	15–20%
Target:		25% (minimum)	55%	20%

1500-Calorie Plan for the Transition Phase

Meal Time	When	What	Calories
	Breakfast	2 scoops of protein meal-replacement powder with 8 ounces nonfat milk AND one 6-ounce container nonfat yogurt (90)	360
	Mid-morning snack	1 serving of fruit AND 1 piece light string cheese or ¼ cup low fat cottage cheese	Up to 50 +50–70
	Lunch	2 scoops of meal-replacement powder with 8 ounces water AND 3 ounces lean meat, fish or chicken	186 +150
	Mid-afternoon snack	1 serving of fruit AND 1 iMetabolic protein bar	Up to 60 +150–160
	Dinner	4 ounces lean meat, fish or chicken 1 serving of vegetables with 1 teaspoon oil/butter or a salad with spray dressing. **or** 1 Lean Cuisine®, Smart Ones®, Healthy Choice® prepared meal	200 + 60 + 36 no more than 400 calories
	Evening snack	1 scoop of protein meal-replacement powder with 4 ounces nonfat milk	135

- Remember, you are responsible for tracking your total intake. You need to maintain accurate accounting of your fruit and vegetable intake so you know exactly what each choice you make represents in caloric value. *Mix and match your options so that you eat no more than 1,500 calories a day.*
- You may swap lunch and dinner and have the prepared meal at lunch instead if desired.
- You may have the protein bar in whichever of the three snack slots you prefer. Still only one a day.
- Take one multivitamin every day.
- Continue to drink a minimum of eight glasses of water daily.

COSTS

Cost is an important factor when considering which weight-loss plan to follow–and the costs of some plans can be surprising to some people. I've found it helpful to give my patients a look at some of the costs they will incur depending on the weight-loss plan they select.

Here's a breakdown to give you some ideas of what to expect.

Six-Month Cost Comparison of Low-Calorie Diets (LCDs)

Optitrim®	$2,580
HMR Modified	$2,549
iMetabolic	$1,860

Cost estimated, based upon a six-month treatment period. iMetabolic program includes daily multivitamins.

Accurate as of date of publication

7 • PHASE TWO: TRANSITION

*Take care of your body with steadfast fidelity. The soul
must see through the eyes alone, and if they are dim, the
whole world is clouded.*

~ Goethe

TRANSITION AND LEAN BODY MASS

Loss of muscle mass diminishes strength, endurance, and your sense of
well-being, along with tone and body mechanics. But even if you could
live with that, there's another component to losing muscle mass—it makes
it harder to keep the weight off in the future. In fact, it makes future
weight gain almost inevitable, which is the last thing you want.

> Keep in mind that lean body mass correlates
> directly to your resting, or basal, metabolic rate.
> The more lean body mass you carry on your body,
> the higher your resting metabolic rate and the
> easier you will find Transition and Maintenance.
> Having said this, all future success in Maintenance
> leads toward the adoption of a physical activity
> routine that becomes a long-term habit.

If you've lost too much lean muscle mass during the Induction phase,
the Transition phase could be a problem for you; you may find that it's
easier to gain the weight back when you resume eating, even though you
consume fewer calories each day than you did before you started your
weight-loss program.

In addition, as you enter the Transition phase of your weight loss, you will have already lost most, if not all, of the weight you wanted to lose. As a result, the weight you continue losing every week is probably slowing. Happily, if you've been preserving your lean body mass as you lost the weight and working to build more muscle rather than just maintaining, you're now a more efficient fat-burning machine. Even though your weight loss has slowed, you're still burning calories–and at a higher rate than you would be if you'd lost lean mass as well as fat.

Studies have shown that people who maintain lean body mass during the course of a diet are significantly more likely to succeed at maintaining a healthier weight and at avoiding weight regain in the long run than those who do not preserve their lean body mass. You want to be one of those people who maintains muscle mass during your low-calorie diet. The benefits of doing so really make that 30-minutes-a-day workout worthwhile.

TRANSITION AND EXERCISE

A good low-calorie weight-loss program is structured to help you maintain lean body mass in two ways. First (and, by far, the most important), it incorporates exercise. It's not possible to overemphasize the importance of this. State-of-the-art programs like the one at iMetabolic involve regular exercise as a key component for anyone enrolling in the medically supervised program.

Exercise is especially important during the Transition phase. Even after losing 40 pounds, exercise can be daunting for the severely overweight. Some of our clients have developed some pretty significant degenerative disk disease, which can limit their mobility and make exercise painful and unappealing. I've had several patients over the years whose bad hips, knees, or backs made it difficult for them to even take a walk. But a creative exercise coach will find a way for each person in the program to incorporate daily exercise, and that coach will work with the program doctors to make certain that exercise is safe. For those clients who find land-based exercise too difficult or painful, for example, swimming and other forms of water-based exercise allows them to work out while avoiding injury or pain.

MINDLESS CONSUMPTION OF CALORIES

As you transition out of your 90-day Induction weight-loss plan and back into real life and real food, you're also transitioning from your old, not-so-healthy behaviors to new, healthier behaviors. In addition to adding exercise to your daily life and learning how to resist the allure of random food offerings, you're also looking out for negative behaviors that can creep up on you if you're not paying attention.

Mindless eating is no more or less than the name implies. It's not a big medical mystery; it's what happens when you fall back into familiar behavior patterns. Mindless eating takes place whenever you eat something without having deliberately intended to, without being fully aware of the food you're eating, and without being aware, really, that you're even eating it.

> Mindless eating most often occurs when we are somewhat disconnected from what we are doing. Be on the defensive against mindless eating while working, watching television, driving, working on the computer, reading, or performing other distracting activities. The best defense is to set boundaries on where you permit yourself to eat. Limit your eating to the kitchen or dining room table, your workplace lunch room, and other appropriate places, if any. Don't fall prey to this habit that we've all seemed to develop.

Have you ever made the commitment, first thing in the morning, that today you're going to eat healthy; eat less; stick to your diet—and then, at some point during the day, you realize you've just eaten a jelly doughnut or a handful of jellybeans or had a sugary soda? This is habit. You're moving through your day the way you usually do because somewhere in that day you forgot your goal. Most of us have a pattern to our days, and if your pattern has involved taking a handful of M&Ms from the office candy dish, eating a bagel during the morning meeting, or having that energy-producing soda after lunch, it's easy to find yourself mid-swallow with your brain screaming, "What are you doing?"

One reason it's called mindless eating is that being aware, or *mindful,* can help you defuse this behavior. If your mindless eating takes place at the office, start being aware of what makes you get up in the first place and leave your desk or work station to find the food. Are you making a trip somewhere to do something that involves your job? Then stay focused on it and skip the part of the trip that involves dipping into the food.

What is happening is that habit has produced triggers. Getting up to go to the copier is the trigger for those M&Ms. Sitting in a meeting is a trigger for bagels. Only mindfulness and awareness can nullify the triggers of your habits.

If you find you fall prey to mindless eating on weekends, what activities can you n place that will interrupt your habit of mindlessly wandering into the kitchen and grazing? Can you put barriers in front of the fridge or pantry that prompt you to "come to" and realize what you're about to do? Better yet, would anyone suffer terribly if the only things available to graze on were no more harmless than vegetables and fruit (or protein powder and protein bars)?

If evening's your downfall, I suggest you find activities other than watching television. If you have some favorite shows you love to watch—and most of us do—make certain you're substituting some behavior for the mindless eating you're used to doing while you watch them. Work out with hand weights. Ride an exercise bike. Pace. Take up knitting. Pet the cat. Just don't eat.

One thing that I've come to learn, over the years of helping people lose weight, is that afternoon and evening downfalls often occur because of things that we've done incorrectly earlier in the day. Missing or skipping meals or eating foods with too many simple carbohydrates during the day often cause cravings to surface later in the day, after we are home and relaxed a bit. I've had more than one patient refer to this as the time his "monster" comes out or the "bad" guy surfaces. By not eating correctly earlier in the day, we feed this "monster" or "bad guy," who can come out later and cause problems. Be aware of this and stick to your mission.

Mindless Evening Eating Patterns
1. Snacking on food that's been left on plates while cleaning the table and putting dishes in the dishwasher.
2. "Cleaning up" the food to be stored–neatening edges, trimming so it looks pretty, and eating what you cut off.
3. Eating out of boredom while doing basic chores.
4. Watching television and eating mindlessly. This is one of the top ways to gain unhealthy pounds–it just seems natural for the hand that isn't using the remote to rise and fall to your mouth.

If you routinely stop to pick up a newspaper at the corner convenience store and, as part of that routine, you grab a soda or a candy bar as well, make yourself aware of that behavior and deliberately change it. If you must get something "extra," buy a calorie-free beverage. When you go to the movie theater, the smell of popcorn is pervasive and oh, so appealing. That's a trigger—you automatically assume a movie means popcorn. It doesn't. A movie means entertainment. Popcorn means additional unnecessary calories.

Take some time to learn your own mindless eating triggers and you'll be on your way to becoming mindful and overcoming these behaviors. Take out your journal and write down the triggers you know about. Then take a few days to practice being mindful. Note when, exactly, you reach for unwanted calories. Make a note of any trigger that seems to cause you to want to eat. Finally, work on coming up with alternative ways of handling those triggers and avoiding the calories.

Peak performance begins with your taking complete responsibility for your life and everything that happens to you.

~ Brian Tracy

Mindless eating isn't completely your fault. It takes a while to reprogram the pathways of the brain, so if your physical pathway from one part of your job to another takes you by the candy dish or the soda machine and you've always stopped and had a soda or a handful of something that tastes good, it's going to take vigilance on your part to relearn these behaviors. Don't beat yourself up if you slip by accident and find yourself mid-bite—just make plans to prevent it in the future, maybe by rerouting your trip to avoid the land mines.

Wasted Calories

As you become more mindful of your calorie consumption, you'll become more aware of the calories you take in that are not really very worthwhile. These are *wasted calories*—not in the usual sense of waste going in the garbage, but wasted in the sense that you used up your valuable quota of calories on food that didn't taste all that good and wasn't all that enjoyable. Don't waste calories! Make every calorie count by making it a calorie you truly wish to eat and a food that tastes truly wonderful. Otherwise, don't even bother.

8

∙
∙
∙

Phase Three: Maintaining Success

You've worked hard to get to this point. However, long-term weight loss means finding a way of continuing those diet, exercise, and behavior changes that brought your weight down. If you are able to maintain weight loss for a two-year period, you are very likely to have reached permanent weight loss and a new set point. However, I highly recommend that you keep attending support groups, continue weighing in, and continue working hard at this goal of maintaining a healthy weight. Don't become complacent!

Up to this point, most of your dietary intake has been under the control of your program team through the use of medically formulated weight-loss products. Now comes the time when you begin to introduce life-long change through your choices of food intake. If you look back at the principles you learned during Induction, you'll see you've been concentrating on increasing or maintaining healthy sources of protein in your diet, cutting back on fats–primarily because that allows you to easily cut back on calories–and limiting the number of carbohydrates you eat. Continuation of these dietary changes is necessary if the weight you lost is to stay off.

It's important to stick to the following guidelines; however, if you find yourself in a situation where these food choices are not available, then just do the best you can with portion control. Take time every day to plan your day so that you do not find yourself in a position where you have no options.

You're not going to go the rest of your life without ever eating another carbohydrate. There are times you're going to compromise and eat less than perfectly. There are times you're going to throw caution to the wind and eat the foods you love. You're human! This doesn't mean that you've blown all that hard work and should give up. Cut yourself some slack. Recognize that it was a one-time celebration or that you've encountered a problem with your eating–was it mindless eating that led to the slip? Mental hunger? Learn from your mistakes and move on. If you find you're struggling, go back to the meal-replacement shakes and bars for a while.

If you find you can't get your diet back under control, you might want to check in with your doctor or your program. There may be some tips and tricks you can add that will get you back on the weight-loss or weight-maintenance track.

Avoid Regaining Unwanted Pounds

I know it will come as no surprise if I tell you that the best way to avoid rebound weight gain is to never allow those pounds access to your body. If you never again gain the weight, and if you continue to lose if you're not quite at your ultimate goal weight now, you won't have to do this again. Think about what that means–a healthy, happy future without the medical complications and just plain unpleasantness of the extra weight.

That joy carries with it the need for vigilance. You need to be aware every day for the rest of your life. Aware of what? Of how happy you are, for one thing. Of how good your body feels at a lower weight. You need to be aware of the exercise you enjoy and the exercise you don't enjoy but do anyway.

A vigorous five-mile walk will do more good for an unhappy but otherwise healthy adult than all the medicine and psychology in the world.

~ Paul Dudley White

And you need to be constantly aware of what you're eating and drinking. Food isn't something you're going to take for granted in the future. Mindless eating is a thing of the past. You've taken responsibility for your life and health and weight into your own hands–why would you ever let that go?

Success is the sum of small efforts, repeated day in and day out.

~ Robert Collier

I have struggled with my weight since birth. I started my first weight loss plan at the tender age of ten. Part of what I came to realize at iMetabolic, is that I am an emotional eater. Emotions in all aspects of my life would trigger poor eating habits until I was 363 pounds. At this point, I was basically unable to walk across a parking lot or even able to handle my eight hour workday.

I was in the worst black hole, feeling more and more depressed. I came to the realization that my weight was holding me back from living a great life. One day, a card came in the mail from iMetabolic so I decided to make an appointment for a consultation. From the very beginning, the staff provided me the *tools to achieve what I thought was never possible. I met with a health coach every week, I also interacted with a physician to gain the medical interaction necessary to begin and monitor my journey, an exercise physiologist to best understand what I needed to do from an exercise perspective, and then most importantly, I met periodically with a psychologist who really helped me sort out everything that was holding me back. I have to say that I feel better than I ever have from both an emotional and physical perspective.*

While my journey is not totally complete, I have been able to lose in excess of 100 pounds over the course of 13 months. I just want to tell everyone that iMetabolic and the approach they prescribed provides all the tools for one to succeed. I can honestly say that, at this point, there are no obstacles standing in my way of living life to its fullest.

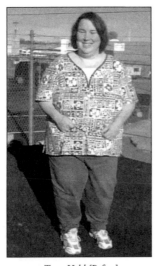

Tracy Held [Before]

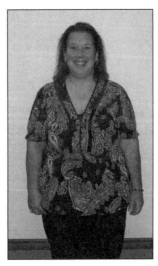

Tracy Held [After]

MAINTAINING YOUR CALORIES

Try looking at your weekly food intake as a *budget* of calories. You have a fixed number, so you want to stay within, and maybe even under, your limit if you're still working on weight loss. Small changes that reduce your daily caloric intake help to prevent weight gain over the course of a year, and they might help you to lose even more weight, if that's what you want. Below are some tips to help you reduce your calorie intake. The more tips you implement, the more calories you cut from your diet.

1. Choose fruit instead of juice: A medium orange has 60 calories, while a cup of orange juice contains 110 calories. Go for the fruit instead. (Calories saved: 50 per day. Weight saved: up to 5 pounds per year.)

2. Downsize your bagel: A mini bagel has only 80 calories, while a regular, medium-sized bagel contains 240 calories– and a typical large bagel has a whopping 350 calories. (Calories saved: 160–270 per day. Weight saved: up to 16–28 pounds per year.)

3. Wrap it up: Have a 10-inch, 110-calorie tortilla instead of a medium, 240-calorie bagel. (Calories saved: 130 per day. Weight saved: up to 13 pounds per year.)

4. Choose light cream cheese: One ounce (two tablespoons) of light cream cheese contains 60 calories, while an ounce of regular cream cheese contains 100 calories. (Calories saved: 40 per day. Weight saved: up to 4 pounds per year.)

5. Go Canadian: Have Canadian bacon, at 90 calories for two slices, instead of regular bacon, at 250 calories for two slices. (Calories saved: 160 per day. Weight saved: 16 pounds per year.)

6. Add the real thing to your yogurt: One cup of fruit-flavored low-fat yogurt contains 230 calories. Instead, have one cup of plain, low-fat yogurt with 1/2 cup of fresh fruit, which totals 180 calories–plus you get the extra benefit of fiber from the fruit. (Calories saved: 50 per day. Weight saved: up to 5 pounds per year.) Better yet, try Dannon Light & Fit™–only 80 calories.

7. Make the mayo light: Replace that tablespoon of regular mayonnaise, which contains 90 calories, with a tablespoon of light mayonnaise, which has only 50 calories. (Calories saved: 40 per day. Weight saved: up to 4 pounds per year.)

8. Spray it: Instead of using a tablespoon of butter or margarine to coat your skillet, use nonstick cooking spray. (Calories saved: 90 per day. Weight saved: up to 10 pounds per year.)

9. Lighten up on butter and margarine: Regular butter or margarine contains 100 calories per tablespoon; light butter or margarine has only 50. (Calories saved: 50 per day. Weight saved: up to 5 pounds per year.)

10. Season up: Instead of a tablespoon of butter or margarine, which contains 100 calories, use herbs to season your vegetables and other foods. (Calories saved: 100 per day. Weight saved: up to 10 pounds per year.)

11. Creamy options: Trade in your nightly half cup of full-fat ice cream for a "light" or reduced-fat version. (Calories saved: 130 per day. Weight saved: up to 13 pounds per year.)

12. Cone down: Choose a small sugar cone to hold your scoop of ice cream instead of a waffle cone–or, better, yet, skip the cone altogether. (Calories saved: 40–100 per day. Weight saved: up to 4–10 pounds per year.)

13. Choose canned fish packed in water: A six-ounce can: A 6-ounce can of chunk light tuna stored in oil has 275 calories. Packed in water, it has only 150 calories. (Calories saved: 125 per day. Weight saved: up to 13 pounds per year.)

14. Lower the fat in your cottage cheese: Have a half cup of 1-percent cottage cheese instead of the 4-percent, full-fat version. (Calories saved: 40 per day. Weight saved: up to 4 pounds per year.)

15. Starching down: So long, starch: Cut your normal, 1/2-cup serving of rice or pasta in half. (Calories saved: 45–60 per day. Weight saved: up to 5–6 pounds per year.

16. Lighten your coffee: Use two tablespoons of whole milk rather than tablespoons of half-and-half. (Calories saved: 20 per day. Weight saved: up to 2 pounds per year.)

17. Make baking healthier: Replace half of the fat in a recipe with applesauce. Per 1/2 cup, applesauce contains 90 calories, but butter or margarine contains a whopping 810 calories. (Calories saved: 720 calories per 1/2 cup/a whopping 75 pounds annually)

18. Slim your soda: Replace that 12-ounce can of sugary soda with a can of calorie-free soda or another calorie-free beverage. (Calories saved: 150 per day. Weight saved: up to 16 pounds per year.)

19. Chow on the right chips: Instead of a small, 2-ounce bag of regular chips, go for a 2-ounce bag of baked chips. (Calories saved: 70 per day. Weight saved: up to 7 pounds per year.)

20. Go fresh: Instead of a half cup of dried fruit, such as raisins, choose a piece or a half cup of fresh fruit. (Calories saved: 190 per day. Weight saved: up to 20 pounds per year.)

21. Vary your chocolate options: Instead of having a 1.5-ounce, 225-calorie chocolate bar, enjoy a 160-calorie cup of chocolate milk or an 85-calorie half cup of fat-free chocolate pudding. (Calories saved: 65–140 per day. Weight saved: up to 6–14 pounds per year.)

22. Ah, nuts: One ounce of nuts (about 23 almonds, 18 medium cashews, 18 to 22 mixed nuts, or 15 to 20 pecan halves) contains 160 to 200 calories. That's a lot of calories for a very little amount of food—so skip them. (Calories saved: 160–200 per day. Weight saved: up to 16–21 pounds per year.}

23. Cheers: Drink a can or bottle of light beer instead of the regular kind. (Calories saved: 30 per day. Weight saved: up to 3 pounds per year.)

24. Wine Not?: Drink 4 ounces of wine instead of 12 ounces of beer. (Calories saved: 50 per day. Weight saved: up to 5 pounds per year.)

25.   Go light on syrup: Two tablespoons of regular syrup contains 110 calories, compared to only 50 calories for light syrup. (Calories saved: 60 per day. Weight saved: up to 6 pounds per year.)

26.   Cut the juice: Have a half cup of orange juice instead of a full cup. (Calories saved: 55 per day. Weight saved: up to 6 pounds per year.)

27.   Leave it behind: Leave the last few bites on your plate. You don't have to finish it all if you're already full. Practice this regularly and you'll find it easier to leave half of your restaurant meal for the doggie bag. (Calories saved: varies. Weight saved: varies.)

Make an effort to use at least one tip each day to help prevent a progressive weight creep over the years. By making little changes like these, you can subtly push the numbers on the scale in the right direction. See how many other calorie-saving ideas you can come up with. (For more tips, take a look at another book of mine–*Doctor's Orders: 101 Medically Proven Tips for Losing Weight*.

Comforting Facts About Comfort Foods

Here's the good news: you don't have to give up everything you love forever. Food associations from childhood can last a lifetime. The dynamics of family eating patterns and the comfort of your own favorite foods have been with you for years. You can overcome these patterns and learn new ones if you remain mindful while eating and determined to stay the course of your weight loss and your new life.

Just because you've lost weight and you're working hard to maintain that healthy weight loss, it doesn't mean that you can't ever have these foods again. In fact, swearing off anything you love *forever* is a recipe for disaster.

Although comfort foods are often unhealthy food choices–most people turn to sweets, salty snack foods, or soft, warm foods like puddings or pastas rather than being comforted by a lean chicken breast–once you've reached the Maintenance phase of your program, you should be able to indulge in some of your comfort foods by making a few small changes.

Cut portions. Rather than a slab of chocolate cake, have a sliver. Rather than a pint of ice cream, have a single serving. In addition to cutting portions, try replacing unhealthy comfort foods with better, but still comforting, choices. Instead of that serving of ice cream, try a serving of frozen yogurt.

The chains of habit are generally too small to be felt until they are too strong to be broken.

~ Samuel Johnson

Eating with Satisfaction

If you want to really enjoy a special dinner out or a special menu you're planning, try just having a very light lunch (maybe a 150-calorie protein bar or shake, for example). By the time you sit down to that special dinner, that first bite will taste like sheer heaven.

What makes the food taste so much better? Even if the food is beautifully prepared by a wonderful chef, it will taste particularly special because you're honestly hungry. You're eating out of true hunger, not emotional or mental hunger; you're not eating just because it's dinner time.

Take advantage of this hunger to really enjoy your food. Remember, you're eating for quality, not quantity. Whether it's a lovingly cooked Thanksgiving dinner or an exquisitely prepared meal at a three-star restaurant, slow down and enjoy every bite.

Even on a special evening, don't change your weight-loss program dietary guidelines. Keep your dinner small and low in carbs, fat, and calories. Examine the texture and feel of your food. Note the sensation and richness of the flavors in your mouth. Breathe in the delicious aromas. Enjoy every sensation, and eat more slowly than usual. Make the pleasure last.

Afterward, ask yourself if you didn't enjoy this dinner more than most. Don't let yourself feel deprived just because you didn't stuff yourself silly. Hunger and the yearning to be completely filled up aren't important. Quite the contrary: for someone who is overweight, these are primal drives that need to be ignored and controlled. Redefine pleasure as more than just satiety. It's time for you to decide that you're in charge of your body and desires–that they don't control you–and to concentrate on the satisfaction of enjoying every bite of food rather than eating too much of it.

Now try approaching all your meals this way: come to the table honestly hungry; eat slowly; and get the maximum pleasure out of the best foods you can eat. It won't take long before you become very choosy about the foods you select to fuel your body and the care with which you prepare them. You'll enjoy your food more, you'll pay attention to what you're eating, and you'll lose weight and become healthier. The only thing you'll lose is excess weight.

Try this exercise

Cut your lunches in half for the next week. Every day, eat half a sandwich and half of the fruit or other foods that come with it. If dessert is part of your normal lunch, skip it. Then, every night, prepare dinner with attention to detail and the best ingredients you have. Eat slowly, savor every bite, and see if you don't get more satisfaction from these dinners than you usually do.

Win or lose; only I hold the key to my destiny.

~ Elaine Maxwell

WAGING WAR ON WEEKENDS

Regardless of your work schedule, you probably have a couple of un-structured days every week when you can catch up on sleep, run errands, play outside, enjoy the company of friends and family, and just plain not adhere to a strict schedule.

Weekends can also make it harder to stay on your weight-loss or maintenance program. Research has shown that Americans between the ages of 19 and 50 take in, on average, 173 more calories per weekend day than they do on weekdays. Over the course of a year, that adds up to nearly 27,000 extra calories (nearly eight pounds annually). Studies also show that most of these extra calories come from alcohol and fat. Mondays are difficult enough for many people to face; it's even worse if they're accompanied by feelings of guilt or remorse about weekend weight gain.

One way to defeat weekend weight gain is to keep active. If your ideal weekend doesn't involve your weekday workouts, try something different—such as hiking, biking, kayaking, swimming, or even walking briskly through the mall—just to make certain you're getting in a period of actual timed movement. If you also remain mindful of burning more calories than you take in, you can stay on top of weekend weight gain and even lose weight over the weekend.

Many of the tips you've already learned will help with the weekend weight war. For example:

- Eat breakfast, and make sure that it contains a lot of protein. Breakfast gets your metabolic motor running and keeps you from being very hungry later on, when you might otherwise binge or eat impulsively.

- Don't overlook your protein-oriented snacks at least twice per day. This is critically important to maintaining your metabolic efficiency.
- If you're planning dinner out, don't starve yourself ahead of time; just cut back on some of your calories in the early part of the day in anticipation of enjoying a restaurant meal that contains more calories. If you're starving by the time you get to the restaurant, it's much too easy to order too much food and to overeat.
- Have a protein shake or bar prior to going to dinner. This will help to take the edge off any hunger you have and will allow you to better control your eating.
- Avoid alcohol. Alcohol is full of empty calories that are stored as fat, and alcohol's ability to lower your inhibitions can make it easy to adopt a devil-may-care attitude toward food consumption.
- Dress for success. Elastic-band pants, sweats, or loose clothes– these aren't your friends. Wear clothes that don't expand along with your stomach, and make sure they're tight enough to send a warning signal when you begin to overeat. If your clothes are feeling tighter as the day goes on, stop eating! You'll stay more aware of how much you are eating and gain less weekend weight. As a bonus, you won't have to worry about fitting into your normal clothes on Monday.

SLEEP BETTER

In today's world, many people simply do not get enough sleep[. Research shows that those who are sleep deprived have a harder time fighting off food cravings and temptations. In addition, those who get less than seven hours of sleep a night put their metabolic systems at risk by not giving their hormone levels time to return from their daily highs to a resting baseline. When hormones are elevated, losing or even maintaining weight becomes more challenging. If you're one of those people, and sleep has become an issue for you, here are some tips to help you get your zzz's.

Life is too short to sleep on low-thread-count sheets.

~ Leah Stussy

Sleep Habits

The most common cause of insomnia is a change to daily routine. Common changes involve travel, a change in hours at work, relationship conflict, and disruption of other activities and behaviors. Changes in eating, exercise, leisure, and work patterns can all contribute to sleep challenges.

The most important thing you can do to ensure that you get enough sleep is to develop and maintain good sleep habits.

Do:
- Go to bed at the same time each day (including weekends).
- Get up from bed at the same time each day.
- Get regular exercise daily, preferably in the morning. Getting enough exercise (stretching and aerobic) can lead to restful sleep.
- Get regular exposure to outdoor or bright light, especially in late afternoon.

- Keep the temperature in your bedroom comfortable.
- Keep the bedroom quiet while you're sleeping.
- Keep the bedroom dark enough to let you sleep.
- Use your bed only for sleep and sex.
- Take medications as directed. If you're taking a prescription sleep aid, take it 30 minutes to an hour before bedtime so you're already drowsy when you lie down.
- Incorporate a relaxation exercise into your nightly routine. Try muscle relaxation, visual imagery, a massage, or a warm bath.
- Keep your hands and feet warm. Wear warm socks and mittens or gloves to bed if your feet and hands are cold.

Don't:
- Perform vigorous or strenuous exercise just before going to bed.
- Engage in anxiety-provoking activity before bed, such as playing a competitive game, watching an exciting TV show, or having an important or distressing discussion with a loved one.
- Have caffeine in the evening (coffee, tea, chocolate, soda, and other caffeinated products).
- Read or watch TV in bed.
- Use alcohol to help you sleep.
- Go to bed too hungry or too full.
- Take another person's prescription sleeping pills.
- Take over-the-counter sleeping pills without your doctor's knowledge. Tolerance can develop rapidly with these medications. And diphenhydramine, an ingredient commonly found in over-the-counter sleep medications, can have serious side effects in elderly patients.
- Take daytime naps.
- Attempt to "command" yourself to go to sleep. This only makes mind and body more alert.

If you lie in bed awake for more than 20 or 30 minutes, get up, go into a different room (or a different part of the bedroom), and engage in a quiet activity, such as reading something or watching television, as long as whatever you're reading or watching isn't really exciting. Return to bed when you feel sleepy. Repeat this behavior as many times a night as necessary.

If people were meant to pop out of bed, we'd all sleep in toasters.

- Anonymous

EXERCISE FOR LIFE

By now, you've incorporated exercise into your daily life. It's probably become a habit. You know it helps you to keep your weight down, and you probably know it makes you feel good, as well. You have no reason to stop. So don't. If you want to live, you have to keep moving. That's especially true if you want to live a strong, healthy, happy life.

In order to lose weight, you need to decrease the number of calories you take in or increase the number of calories you burn. Combining the two is the most effective way to lose weight. You burn more calories and you feel better, too. The average American gains approximately one to two pounds a year after age 25, and most people exercise less as they get older. Continuing that cycle will definitely result in weight gain, the loss of lean body mass, and an increase of body fat.

It's never too late to build muscle mass. It's never too late to improve your condition.

SUPPORT GROUPS

I discussed putting together your own homegrown support group during your weight-loss journey–a group made up of your most supportive friends and family members; those people who absolutely supported your plan to change your life for the better by losing the unwanted weight. Or you may have established a group of like-minded people you didn't know all that well in the beginning but whom you now know pretty darn well. Losing weight is hard enough without trying to go it alone and limiting your sources of information and inspiration.

Once you've lost the weight, or some of the weight, and once you're good and thoroughly launched into the new life you've created for yourself, this is no time to go "lone wolf" and try to take the world by storm by yourself. Invite some friends! Once you've lost the weight, you're going to find a variety of new experiences and new pleasures and new joys ahead of you. Whether you're actually *there* already or just coming close to being there, good for you! You've made a major decision–a life-changing choice for health and longevity.

And maybe you'll never have another minute's concern about your weight. I wish that for you. But, in my experience, many people who have lost weight are at risk of regaining it, no matter what map they followed to their destination.

Weight's a tricky thing to lose. It tends to come back. We still face all the stressors that used to lead us to overeat, such as relationship stress, family stress, and work stress. And, all too often, we succeed at losing all the weight we want to, only to find ourselves more hungry than normal and apt to gain back weight more quickly than normal. This often comes from having lost weight without maintaining enough lean body mass; as a result, our bodies have lost some of their ability to burn calories at rest. (You can find your way back to that ability, of course, and even go beyond it, just by increasing your exercise, especially weight-bearing exercise, which will build up your lean muscle mass.) Whatever the cause, it's likely that, at some point, you're going to be confronted with pounds trying to creep back on or that you'll find yourself in a rebound eating situation where, having lost the weight, you realize you really miss the way you used to eat. Or maybe you haven't seen a single pound try to make its way back onto your body–and you're invested in keeping that trend going.

For all these reasons, this is a great time to be in a support group. If you haven't created or joined one yet, I urge you to seek out a group of people who have lost weight or who are in the process of losing weight, whether it's a group that's affiliated with your weight-loss center, a walking group, your own group of supportive friends and family, or a group of new acquaintances you've met at the gym.

A support group is convenient for sharing information about what works and what doesn't. You can exchange healthy recipes and cheer each other up when you're feeling down. You can inspire each other and see each other through tough places like plateaus, when the weight, for no reason whatsoever, just refuses to come off.

Support groups are made up of people with the same goals and dreams as yours. Losing weight is hard. Keeping it off long-term is hard. I know you have the willpower and confidence to do it–but if you have a chance to help others on their journey and let them help you on yours, I urge you to take it.

* *

After struggling with the yo-yo effect of ineffective fad diets for several years, I finally found a weight-loss program that changed my life. In four months, I lost 30 pounds. More important, I learned from the excellent, friendly staff, especially Natasha Mulqueen, my weekly support and information source, how to change my eating and exercise habits for sustained better health. I look great; I feel great. Thanks to all of you at iMetabolic.

Dennis Grundy–lost 30 pounds in 12 weeks

* *

9

· · ·

The Future and the New You

The benefits of changing your life, your diet, your fitness level, and your style of eating are innumerable. It's not just a matter of having better health, a smaller waistline, and a longer life–the best thing is that you have a new you!

THE NEW YOU

One of the amazing things I see over and over again among people who have successfully accomplished their goals of significant long-term weight loss is that they become better people in many ways. I see in them a formula for long-term success that I want to share with you.

The people that I see so frequently in my practice are truly inspiring individuals. Each started a journey at a time in his or her life when he or she was very self-conscious and full of doubt. Each struggled with being overweight for many years and finally decided to act and make changes in a very positive way.

These are people who gathered immense amounts of information on long-term weight loss and chose to move ahead with a program. They committed to vigorous, long-term changes, an exercise regime, nutritional training, different eating habits, and, in some cases, counseling. Each person hung on when the going got tough: they utilized skills and tools, went to support groups, and called friends for additional support. Sometimes they backslid, but they always went forward again. And, eventually, each reached his or her ultimate goal.

All of these people have done something even more amazing. All of them have changed the circumstances of their lives and opened their eyes to new horizons and new opportunities. In many cases, these people began thinking beyond themselves. They looked to other people to share joy and compassion, and they embarked on new careers, new relationships, and new ideas. Simply by figuring out how to change their lives by losing weight, they figured out how to make other meaningful changes, as well.

It has been said that one of the most important characteristics of a person who achieves goals, succeeds in life, and positively affects the lives of others is the ability to truly empathize and communicate with other people. The idea that you might begin to look more at the lives of people around you and care more deeply about them is not only key to your success as a person, but it is also key to your fulfillment as a human being. Helping those around you proves to be one of the most fulfilling of all human activities. That's why I have added it as one more goal for you. I want you to reach that pinnacle of success–the place where you've reached your goals and can start working to help other people reach theirs. Nothing else can be so rewarding.

ADJUSTING TO THOSE AROUND YOU

Accomplishing substantial weight loss–an accomplishment that results in such dramatic improvements to your health–deserves recognition from those around you. Most of the people in your life, who love you and want the best for you, will feel nothing but great joy at your experience and your transformation. They'll encourage you and take an active interest in learning more about the healthy changes you're making. They'll be interested in working out with you, learning about steps they can take to avoid becoming seriously overweight, and find out the actions they can take to help you stay on the straight and narrow.

But not everyone in your life will react favorably. One of the challenges of your successful weight-loss journey is adapting to the changing nature of your relationships with others.

You'd think that losing, say, 100 pounds and keeping it off for good would be seen as a positive transformation by everyone around you. The truth is often different. Losing so much weight can bring other positive changes in your life. Your accomplishment may alter some of your relationships and take you in new directions. You may find yourself involved in new social activities or even in a new career.

Losing so much weight may make you more attractive to others. It's not uncommon, if you've struggled with self-esteem while battling a weight problem, to emerge from weight loss with both a much healthier body and a much healthier attitude. Once you feel better about yourself, you may become more caring and empathetic toward others, which will make you more attractive to other people.

You may start to attract new friends, and some of your new relationships may affect your old relationships. Sometimes people in your life are used to you the way you were, in a certain role you're expected to keep playing.

Many of my patients have told me that, when they'd show up at family reunions, they'd always had the sense that they fulfilled the role as "the overweight aunt" or some other silly stereotype. When they lost the weight, they no longer fit the role that had been assigned them by other people, and this sometimes led to upheaval in their relationships.

Another example I've seen is that of the seriously overweight spouse who loses the weight and becomes a more attractive person, thus creating a perceived threat to the marital relationship.

So this tremendous positive change that will have wonderful, long-term effects on your life may also create some complexities and challenges in your personal relationships. How should you cope with these changes and challenges? There's no simple or easy answer, but there are a few things that may help you as you navigate these waters.

For starters, remind yourself of your own goals. Remember what it is you're setting out to achieve. Look back to the things you wrote down that were and still are so important to you. Remember the huge positive impact you're making on your life, your health, and your longevity.

Don't be deterred from your goals by someone who doesn't understand the importance of what you are doing, thinks that exercise is a waste of time, believes that lots of carbs are good for you, or decides that you're not being a great friend if you won't spend all day eating pizza and cake and watching television together. You have a higher goal. Remind yourself of it. What you're doing is important.

Even if the stressors your friends and family are experiencing seem a little silly to you, remember that those feelings are very real to them. They may not even be aware of these feelings or understand them consciously. Take the time to reassure them that you still love them, that the changes you are making haven't negatively changed who you are inside, and that what you're accomplishing will only improve your long-term relationships with others and allow you to remain in their lives.

Thank friends and family for supporting you on your journey. Tell them how much it matters to you to lose the weight and to lead a healthier, happier life with them. Tell them how much their support has meant and how much you still need it. There's nothing wrong with reassuring loved ones that you're not losing weight simply to be more attractive to other people or to leave friends and family behind. Summarize your most important goals, and remind them that your accomplishments will improve not only your own life and health, but your relationships as well.

And when people are supportive and helpful as you chase your goals, take the time to thank and acknowledge them—doing so is not only kind and responsible, but it also may defuse tensions before they ever fully develop.

GET MOVING

Walking is the easiest way to get started with your daily workout regime. It costs very little, it's safe, and it gets you out of the house or workplace and out into the world. Almost anyone can safely start a walking program and make intentional physical activity part of daily life.

Before you embark on your walking program count the number of steps you normally take each day to get a feel for how much you're already moving. The average American walks between 3,000 and 5,000 steps per day.

STEPS PER DAY	ACTIVITY LEVEL
Fewer than 5,000	Inactive
5,000–7,500	Slightly active
7,500–10,000	Moderately active
10,000–12,500	Active
More than 12,500	Very active

Tips for Walking

- Plan to walk at least 30 minutes five to six days a week.
- If you can't walk 30 minutes at a time at the beginning, go as far as you can comfortably and build up from there.
- If you don't have 30 minutes available at one time, take two 15-minute walks.
- Wear comfortable clothes and shoes.
- Don't overdo it. Rest if you get tired.
- If you're an outdoor walker, have an alternative in mind for bad-weather days.
- Wear a pedometer.
- Track your steps.
- Set goals for increasing your steps.

Step Equivalents for Activities Other Than Walking

ACTIVITY	EQUIVALENT STEPS PER MINUTE:	
	WOMEN	MEN
Cycling	150	180
Downhill skiing	150	180
Cross-country skiing	225	270
Swimming	95	115
Weight lifting	100	120
Yoga	50	60

Tips for Increasing Activity
At Home
- Get up to change the channel rather than using the remote.
- Walk around the house during commercials.
- Exercise in front of the TV rather than just sitting there.
- Pace around the house while talking on the phone.
- If you have stairs in your house, use them—even if you don't need to go to the next floor.
- Make more trips unloading the car after shopping. Carry one bag at a time.
- Get a push lawn mower.
- Rake leaves and sweep sidewalks rather than using a blower.
- Shovel the snow.
- Wash your car in the driveway rather than using a drive-through carwash.
- Walk to the mailbox if your mail is delivered at a central location.
- Take the dog for a walk.
- Play fetch with the dog.
- Don't have a dog? Borrow the neighbor's.
- Play ball with your kids, grandkids, or each other.
- Go for a bike ride.
- Put on your favorite music and dance.
- Energetically clean your house.

Around Town
- Park at the far end of every parking lot. There is tons more parking there anyway.
- Park in one spot and walk to as many errands as you can.
- Return your grocery cart to the return corral or to the store itself.
- Use the stairs instead of elevators or escalators.
- Explore parks and trails you haven't visited.
- Go to community events and walk around.
- Go to the museum.

- Walk around inside the mall. Explore new shopping areas.
- Avoid the drive-through at the bank and at other places. Park far away from the building's entrance and walk in.
- Walk the concourse at the airport rather than taking the people-moving belts.

Around Work
- Park as far away as you can or get off the bus a few stops early and walk the rest of the way.
- Use the stairs whenever possible.
- Get up from your desk every 30 minutes and just move.
- Use your break times to move around the office.
- Keep walking shoes under your desk and walk, jog, or bike on your breaks.
- Find an activity friend for break time.

You need to start somewhere, and the more activity you can include in your days, the more weight you'll lose and the better you'll keep it at bay.

Log everything you can. The more you keep track of, the more you can see at a glance what you're doing–and what you're doing well and what you could be doing better. See appendixes C and D for a walking program and for 100 exercises you can do at home.

Fitness–if it came in a bottle, everybody would have a great body.

~ Cher

PLATEAUS AND RELAPSES

Once you've successfully started to lose the weight, I'm betting you'll find that it's such a good feeling it feels addictive. You'll get up in the morning and note what you've lost since the day before, the week before, or the month before. Watching that weight slide away; seeing that scale react a little less every time—it's amazing. You feel better with every pound you lose, too—stronger; more fit; more confident. Happier. If you were suffering health consequences related to being overweight or obese, you're now experiencing the health benefits of losing those excess pounds.

The extent to which all of that feels wonderful is matched only by the frustration felt when weight loss slows, or even stops, for no reason you can determine.

It's not about whether or not you are knocked down; it's about whether or not you get up.

~ Vince Lombardi

When Reality Bites

If you've been celebrating and living that new life, this isn't the time you want to contemplate what you're going to do if the weight loss slows or stops. But it's better to know ahead of time that plateaus can occur—that weight loss can slow to a crawl or stop—so that you can make plans in advance to handle it.

A weight-loss plateau can happen even if you have altered absolutely nothing from what's been working for you. Even if you're still eating the way you were when you were losing weight. Even if you're still creating an energy deficit every day. Even if you've added exercise to your daily routine and you're moving for at least 30 minutes every day. Even then, a weight-loss plateau can happen, and the weight can just stop coming off.

It's frustrating. It's maddening. It's just unfair.

Don't panic. Plateaus break. It's not permanent, even if it feels permanent. You will start losing weight again–and chances are good that, down the road, you'll eventually hit more plateaus. Weight loss is a balky start-and-stop process with so many internal and external variants that a plateau isn't unusual. What would be unusual is smooth, consistent weight loss that started with a specific number of pounds per week and continued that way to the end.

That said, there are steps you can take to get off the plateau and start losing weight again. I know you didn't plan to just wait it out.

I've seen hundreds of my patients run into plateaus, get frustrated, get motivated and start losing weight again. You will, too. Plateaus are common. Your body is looking for stable ground as you move from one size to another. It was used to being where it was, and you've gone and shaken up the status quo; you've changed things. That was what you were supposed to do, but your body's still wondering what you were thinking. You've gone and created a calorie deficit, and that's made your caveman genes nervous. It's very likely that your body is trying to conserve energy and hoard every calorie it can get its hands on. Until it figures out where this new road is taking it, it doesn't want to keep going down that road.

The thing is, your body will figure things out. It may take time, which I know is frustrating, but you're not just trying to lose weight and see a smaller figure on the scale and a smaller size in the closet. You're changing your entire life. You're fighting for healthy weight loss, a healthy future, and victory in the long-term battle.

Always bear in mind that your own resolution to succeed is more important than any other one thing.

~ Abraham Lincoln

You can do this. There are steps you can take to restart your weight loss today.

1. Look at all the reasons you want to lose weight. It's not just about smaller clothes or a smaller number on the scale; it's also about living longer and being a happier, healthier you.

2. If you haven't yet done so, write down all the reasons you wanted to lose weight. If you were concentrating solely on looking better, start detailing some of the other major benefits, such as lower blood pressure, lower cholesterol, less back and joint pain, better endurance, the end of diabetes, or improved fertility. Write them down. You've been losing weight. You will again. Frustrating as the plateau is, you've already made healthy changes to your life. This is not time to despair.

3. Write down what you're eating and drinking for a few days. Have you made any changes from what was working? Review the pattern of your foods and see if you find evidence of too many carbs or calories or too much fat. Maybe you've begun mindlessly drinking sugared sodas again. Maybe there's something else. Keep a food journal to see whether or not any aspect of your diet has changed.

4. *Change* your diet. If you were using a liquid protein meal-replacement plan for a while, go back to it. If you weren't, consider trying it. A low-calorie diet (using meal-replacement shakes) right now could jump-start your weight loss again.

5. Don't stop eating, especially when it comes to breakfast. Breakfast gets the metabolism revved and running in the morning, and the more protein you can take in, from steak and eggs (hold the hash browns) to protein shakes and bars, the better. This is the

way to go. If some of those carbs, such as cereals, bagels or white toast, have sneaked back into breakfast, send them packing. Tell them to take the plateau with them.

6. Get moving. Even if you're already following an exercise routine, try to squeeze some more physical activity into each day. If you're not exercising, why not? Start now.

7. Don't forget sleep. Remember that you need a minimum of seven hours of quality sleep each night. Cutting corners in this area can definitely help fuel a plateau.

MAKE YOUR WEIGHT LOSS LAST

Whether you've lost 10 pounds or 100, you have a better chance of keeping it off if you change your modus operandi to one that includes healthier habits–and if you keep up those habits after the weight-loss program itself ends.

- Keep weighing yourself on the schedule you've been following. Allow yourself some wiggle room–a three- to five-pound weight gain isn't the end of the world, and you don't need to panic or feel you've failed. Just increase your exercise or curtail your calories for a few days. A little wiggle room also gives you the freedom to eat a few of your favorite foods, which means you won't binge on them.
- Eat small meals at frequent regular intervals. This helps to keep your metabolism burning calories and it keeps you from getting hungry and eating something you shouldn't. I can't stress this enough. The one common thread that I see among nearly every single patient I interact with is that he or she sometimes skips meals. Just remember, that caveman metabolism that we all have is scared to no end by missing meals. This sends the "storage" signals like crazy. Let me repeat, don't skip meals!

- Eat your protein first. During the Induction phase, your diet was largely comprised of protein. Remember, protein and amino acids are the building blocks of lean muscle mass. Protein is very satisfying and it isn't stored in the body as fat. Therefore, it's a good idea to begin each meal by eating the protein. Eat the fats next, and eat the carbs only if you're still hungry.
- Prepackaged foods that claim to be "fat free," "reduced fat," "light," or "diet" are often anything but. The next time you're in a grocery store, check the food labels of some of these "diet" foods; you'll be surprised at how many calories and carbs and how much fat are in them.
- Get rid of your "fat clothes." You don't ever want to wear those again!
- Find a piece of clothing you particularly like in your new size and use it as a marker. The scale may fluctuate, but your clothes should fit the same each time. If your favorite jeans start feeling tight, watch what you're eating and pick up your exercise.
- Buy a copy of *Doctor's Orders: 101 Medically Proven Tips for Losing Weight*. Keep it on your nightstand or at work and incorporate as many of the tips into your daily routine as you possibly can to maintain the weight loss. This book is filled with ideas for weight loss and it may offer some suggestions you've never considered. If nothing else, it certainly offers enough variety to help you keep mixing it up.

I don't want to live in a world where I have to eat sugar-free sugar cookies.
~ *Animal Crossing: Wild World*

9 • The Future and the New You

Take the Power Out of Peer Pressure

The people around you may not understand the struggle that food creates in your life. Friends who are at normal weights or who are underweight may respond with tales of their own binges or misadventures with foods. They may admit to cravings or try to compare their behavior to yours. The underlying message seems to be that we're all just human and that you should relax and enjoy yourself. The best thing you can do for these well-meaning friends is acknowledge their concern and explain the work you've done and are doing, the positive life change you've experienced and are still making, and the best ways that they can help you.

Then again, friends and family may want to test your resolve. They may tease you or goad you. They may fix your favorite high-calorie meals just to see what happens. It's not kind, but it happens. Just stay your course, trust yourself, explain what you're doing (possibly explain *again* what you're doing), and move on. Eventually, they'll come to understand that you mean business.

Unless these are people who don't want you to succeed. I wish I could say there aren't people like that out there, but there are. They may be jealous of your success. They may envy your resolve and your weight loss. Even your thin friends can envy the sense of accomplishment you're getting from pursuing and succeeding at your goals. Your friends who are overweight may feel threatened. While you're losing weight, they may imagine they're losing you and try, either unconsciously or not, to undermine your efforts by offering you food, eating in front of you, or discussing what's going to happen after you've gained it all back–after you've failed. Show them your friendship by sticking through this phase even while you stick to your guns. These people may decide to end the friendship themselves, but it's more likely that they'll eventually come to understand that both the friendship and the weight loss are important to you–and that you both can move to a "new normal" in your relationship together.

Some of the people in your life may become super aware of eating in front of you. These individuals might be afraid of tempting you, or they might worry that you're judging them with every bite they take. Tell your friends to relax–you've made the changes and you're happy with those changes. Your friends are free to carry on as they always have.

Last, some people in your life who aren't changing their eating habits and their lives may consider your diet to be dangerous. They might be afraid that you're starving or that you've become anorexic and, because they care about you, they may try to feed you. Politely refuse, explain that you're fine, and change the subject.

Most of the time your friends and family will and should be supportive. Some of them might even join you once they see the results you're getting. Welcome their participation with open arms–but make sure you understand, even if they don't, that your weight loss is your responsibility and that their weight loss is their responsibility. If your friends and family try and fail, it doesn't mean you will. You've already put in the time, energy, and discipline to succeed.

PLAN AHEAD

How many weight-loss wars are lost because the battle wasn't planned? If your life is busy and complicated and every minute is spoken for, finding time for a healthy meal is challenging. If you're trying to eat six small meals a day, it can be more challenging–how do you do that when you're constantly on the go? Today's world is full of business travel and children's sports events and late meetings and business lunches. How long will it be before you give up on the carefully structured meals and just grab what's there because you're hungry?

It doesn't have to happen at all. Don't leave your food choices to chance. Chance is a terrible diet coach!

And have a backup plan. I keep my car stocked with protein bars and my kitchen and office stocked with protein shakes–because sometimes I can't plan, can't prepare, and can't cook. But this way, I've always got some low-calorie, low-carb foods that I know I can get to before I become an out-of-control, very hungry doctor.

*Those who trust to chance must abide by
the results of chance.*

~ Calvin Coolidge

Tips on Planning Ahead

- Plan your menus a week at a time. Go through each recipe and make sure you have all the ingredients so you're not constantly running back to the store.
- Make a complete grocery list–again, the fewer trips to the store, the fewer chances for an impulse buy.
- Shop around the edges of the store. That's where the produce, meats, and dairy are. Stay away from the center aisles, where the high-calorie, high-carb processed foods are located.
- When grocery shopping, stick to your list. Take advantage of coupons, but only for the allowed foods–you're not saving anything if you pick up foods you're not supposed to eat just because they're on sale. And make certain you're not hungry when you're shopping–your willpower is much stronger if everything doesn't look quite so tempting.
- If you're constantly running late, do as much as you can when you first get home from the store. Separate items into single servings. Prepare salad fixings and store each ingredient in its own container or bag.
- If you tend to rush around in the mornings, take the time to assemble the components of your breakfast and lunch each night. This will help you save time in the mornings, and it will help you to avoid grabbing some packaged or fast-food lunch because you didn't have time to prepare a healthy meal to bring to work.

- Read labels. Know what you're getting. Ingredients are listed in descending order of amounts, so there's more of the first item listed than the next. Pay attention to the numbers of carbohydrates and calories that are in the food you're buying and avoid anything with high-fructose corn syrup, trans fats, and partially hydrogenated oil. Scrutinize the food label of any product that claims to be diet, light, reduced, or low in fat. A "diet" version of a product that has, for example, half the fat as its "regular" version may have twice as much sugar as that original version.

Don't forget to pay attention to serving sizes. A package that looks so small that it can't possibly contain more than one serving may, in fact, contain three or more (as "serving" is defined by the manufacturer). And that list of carbs and calories and everything else only refers to one serving. If they're trying to pull the wool over your eyes, stop and ask yourself why. If the answer is that there's a truckload of calories in a tiny serving, make the decision as to whether or not that food really tastes good enough to waste all those calories on it.

You can repackage foods into your own serving sizes, also. If you are eating individual servings of crackers or snack foods, break them down into the exact portion size for you so you're not fooling yourself when you're hungry and dishing out a snack and taking just a little bit more than you know you should.

STAY COMMITTED

The key to life-changing weight loss is that it begins with life change and change for life. Losing this weight means thinking differently and becoming a different person; a person who is healthier and who thinks about himself or herself and what he or she eats and does–who he or she is–in a different way. Forever. Staying committed to the new you means never giving up on the life changes you have made.

After being injured in a serious accident, I let my weight get out of hand. I have always been very physically active and hard-working, and I served as a volunteer firefighter. My weight gain made these physical activities difficult. I became self-conscious and I was starting to develop high blood pressure.

After hearing an advertisement for Dr. Sasse's center, iMetabolic, I met with the staff. They were very friendly, knowledgeable, and energetic. I decided to give them a go. I started on August 1, 2008. I met with the staff physician, who also was very helpful. Upon using iMetabolic's nutritional education, eating program, and supplements–and by putting in a lot of hard work and discipline–I was able to lose 70 pounds. My body fat is now one quarter of what it was, my fitness level is very high, and my blood pressure is back to a healthy, normal level.

I am a huge numbers guy, and iMetabolic has a body composition machine. We used the machine on a bimonthly basis. I found it very motivating to compare my current results to my previous results and to see that I'd improved on the previous results. I cannot thank iMetabolic and the staff enough.

Robert Shaw–lost 70 pounds

You have to say, "I think that, if I keep working at this and want it badly enough, I can have it."

~ Lee Iacocca

What you've accomplished takes guts and perseverance, tenacity and willpower. A good many people start what you've started; not everyone meets the challenges and triumphs. If you're still on your way, good for you. I have confidence you'll get there. You've learned a lot by reading this book–not just tips and tricks for losing weight, but also information about the metabolic processes that trigger weight gain and weight loss– and you're in a position to apply your knowledge to your own situation. You're light years past where you were when you started.

But I'd like to add right here: You have what it takes *to never have to do this again.* You've lost the weight or you're losing it. You're feeling confident and strong–more confident and stronger with every pound you lose–and that's a great feeling! But, as is true with many challenges, once you've done it? That's enough.

Once the weight is gone, keeping it off must become your number one goal, and there are many challenges to keeping the weight off. Once you've been overweight and lost the weight, vigilance and mindfulness are required for the rest of your happier, healthier, longer life. It's up to you to keep feeling as good as you do now–or even better. Remember and adopt the adage: *If it is to be, it's up to me!*

And there's another component you may choose to include in your life. Others may have helped you along the way, from the people in your support group to your friends and family who supported your goals to change your life for the better.

Now it's your turn.

GIVING BACK

Once you've lost the weight, or lost a significant portion of it, look around and ask yourself who helped you along the way. Maybe friends and co-workers went out of their way to eat healthy foods around you and to encourage your efforts. Maybe you were in a great support group with members who were willing to share all their information. Maybe you had a great team at a weight-loss center. Whatever your individual circumstances, if there were people who helped you along the way, now it's your turn to give back.

Giving back is satisfying. It means that you've achieved your goal (or are well on your way to achieving it) and that you are now in a position to help others. And there are many ways to do so. You can give back in support groups by sharing information as well as your ideas and experiences. You can encourage friends who are just starting out on the same journey you just completed. You can be the person in the office who sets up walking groups for breaks and lunch hours. In northern Nevada, one of the groups I helped form, the Obesity Prevention Foundation (www.obesitypreventionfoundation.org), sends experts into schools and works to help prevent childhood obesity.

Whatever path you choose, I urge you to find some way to share your good fortune with others. You'll feel great as you watch them start to meet their goals–and, as a little added incentive, every time you explain the principles of weight loss to someone else, you reinforce your own knowledge and desire to achieve your weight-loss and weight-maintenance goals.

The Helping Angels program that we run through Western Bariatric has enriched the lives of hundreds of people and promises to enrich those of thousands more in the years to come. The Helping Angels are patients who have already gone through the process of weight loss, made the commitment to health, and transformed their lives. Now they provide support and assistance to those who are coming along behind them.

Helping Angels contribute in support groups by encouraging new members to talk about hurdles yet to be crossed. They've been a major source of inspiration to our patients who are just embarking upon the weight-loss journey and to those who are struggling with the process.

If there are support groups in your area, and if you want to encourage others the way others encouraged you during your journey, I urge you to contact those groups and ask if you can participate from your unique vantage point–that of someone who has already succeeded.

However, you don't have to be in a formal program to encourage others as they strive to achieve their weight-loss goals. You can lead by example.

When eating with friends and family, let them see what you're ordering at restaurants (leaner, more wholesome food) and how much you're eating (or leaving on your plate). Share your knowledge of nutrition. Explain why you're working out and the importance of building and maintaining lean body mass.

If you have children or grandchildren, one of the greatest gifts you can give them is a sound foundation of good nutrition and healthy eating habits. OK, let me get my soapbox out for a minute: Our kids are going to have the most significant weight challenges that have ever been seen by any generation. It's already a big issue. It's not only up to us to set a good example, but it's also our responsibility to enlighten our youth with knowledge that we learn regarding how we behave and adapt to the abundance of food that we now have available.

If you have friends or family members who are interested in what you're doing or who have expressed jealousy or envy over the changes you've made in yourself, offer to share everything you know. Offer to be a support person; the one who can be called when the desire to overeat or eat the wrong things is running high.

You may want to take your efforts of support to another level by working on preventing and treating obesity at a school, community, or state level. There is nothing to stop you. Let people know you're willing to be there for them and that you're willing to share what you've learned. Let them know how happy you are and how much better you've felt since you lost the weight. It's a gift you can give others that can't be matched.

And, if the others aren't ready to make those changes or follow in your footsteps, be patient. Give them time. Continue your own weight loss or maintenance and be the best example you can be. Or consider joining forces with an organization such as the Obesity Prevention Foundation or some other like-minded entity that seeks to educate the masses about how to behave in a world of ever-increasing opportunities to overeat.

9 • The Future and the New You

Start Today

You hold in your hands the keys to successful weight loss and positive change in your life. Don't wait another minute to begin. Don't wait for more advice; don't wait until Monday morning Don't wait to become completely organized or to have just the right timing or until other things have settled down in your life or until you read the next book or until all the stars are properly aligned. Start today. (This is true for any endeavor you want to undertake.)

> *To accomplish great things, we must not only act, but also dream; not only plan, but also believe.*
>
> ~ Anatole France

So often, when we think about a change we'd like to make in our lives, we envision the change and we envision our new selves–and still we hesitate. We hesitate because we haven't clearly crystallized and written down our specific goals for change. Or because we don't have a clear plan or path ahead of us for making that change. Or because we view the change as too big and too daunting, so we don't take the first step. Or because we don't feel that the timing is quite right somehow or that we don't feel quite ready. Or because we believe there are other impediments in our lives or among our friends or family members.

But you've pushed past those doubts and fears. You've envisioned the goal. You've identified and written down your specific goals for a healthier weight and a healthier life. You have committed yourself to making a life change. And now you have the tools you need to capture success. I've spent my entire medical career helping people lose weight, and I've laid out for you all the specific, tried-and-true steps of a highly effective program for losing weight and changing your life. The program builds on proven techniques and valuable lessons learned from helping thousands of people succeed at losing weight at one of the premiere medically based weight-loss centers in the world.

The time to start is now. You won't be able to accomplish the whole journey in one step, but you can't accomplish any of the journey without taking that first step. So take that first step today.

Believe and act as if it were impossible to fail.
~ Charles F. Kettering

NO ONE CAN DO IT FOR YOU

Remember, no one else can make true changes in your life. You're responsible for making the choices and changes that improve your energy level, your sense of well-being, and your health. And the greatest gift you can give yourself is to make positive changes to your life through life-changing weight loss.

It's a gift you deserve. You deserve a better life, better health, and all the other benefits that come with these positive changes you're making, including better social and financial rewards, improved self-esteem, and more happiness because you have a healthier, more physically fit body.

This really is a do-it-yourself project in every sense of the word. No one else is going to make the decisions for you that you're making on a daily basis–skipping dessert; limiting or eliminating your consumption of alcohol; turning down French fries and sugared sodas; refusing chips and crackers. You're the one deciding to wear a pedometer in the morning to chart your steps and hit your goal of 8,000 or 10,000 or 15,000 steps for the day. You're the one reading labels, tracking calories, and creating a calorie deficit, and you're the one lacing up your walking shoes and heading out the door.

You're doing this yourself, *for yourself.* It's the most important thing you could possibly choose to do.

The flip side is also true. You have to claim responsibility if you succumb to temptation; if you order from the dessert menu or binge in private or accept *just one bite* from those helpful bakers in your life. You're the one choosing to skip the day's exercise, and you're the one choosing whether or not to look for other active ways to burn calories and get healthier. If you start regaining the weight and don't take positive, active steps to stop it by revisiting your doctor, creating a calorie deficit, going on a short-term meal-replacement diet, or listening to your supporters, then you're the one who bears complete responsibility for your choices.

It's both exciting and alarming. You get to choose. You choose how you live your life.

Carpe diem.

~ Horace

(Latin: Seize the day)

199

Appendixes

APPENDIX A: BMI (BODY MASS INDEX) AND THE RISK OF TYPE 2 DIABETES

Type 2 diabetes has become one of the most important health problems in our country today and indeed, around the world. It is not only affecting adults and older people, as we used to see in the past, but it is affecting children. Increasingly we are seeing kids in adolescence develop severe type 2 diabetes and the complications of it. Type 2 diabetes is really difficult, not just because living with it every day means taking medicines and monitoring blood sugar, but, in many cases, it means taking insulin shots. In reality, it is really a lifestyle change and it is something that people have to live with that is not an easy thing. Even worse than that, type 2 diabetes, over the years, will lead to other health problems like early heart attacks, blindness, kidney failure or amputations. These are issues that none of us wants for any of our friends, loved ones or children.

Treating type 2 diabetes has become one of the highest priorities for all of us in medicine and healthcare. To gain some visibility, at the root of this condition, we have to recognize that most cases of type 2 diabetes stem from weight gain and obesity. If these conditions are not the direct cause, then both are certainly a major contributor. In fact, research shows there is a direct correlation between BMI (Body Mass Index) and type 2 diabetes. Females are more than twice as at risk as males. At a BMI of 25, females have an eight times greater risk of getting type 2 and males a two times greater risk than either population at a BMI level of 22. The further out one moves on the BMI scale, the more the risk escalates to the point that at a 35 BMI, females are in excess of 90 times more at risk and males over 40 times more so than their counter parts at a 22 BMI.

The good news is, though, that we can cure type 2 diabetes. We can control it and in many cases, we can eliminate it with proper treatment. The proper treatment in this case is clearly aiming at weight loss. Most medicines to treat type 2 diabetes are really only aimed at controlling the disease or controlling the blood sugar number. They are not really affecting the root cause. Even worse than that, many of the medicines that are used to treat diabetes actually have a terrible side effect of causing additional weight gain.

To really get to the core cause of this terrible disease, we have to focus on weight loss. Medically supervised weight loss program like the iMetabolic Weight-Loss Program or other physician-supervised programs work very well to combat this issue in particular. At iMetabolic, we have recently had several people who have reduced their weight significantly to the point that their blood sugar levels have normalized and they have told us "My diabetes is gone now" and, their endocrinologists confirm this as well. Therefore, these patients do not have to take medicines anymore, period as long as they keep their weight in check. It is a matter of helping that person get engaged in the right program with the right doctor and making it happen.

APPENDIX B: BODY MASS INDEX

Body mass index (BMI) is a reliable indicator of body fat for most people. It's calculated based on height and weight–it's not a direct measure of body fat percentage–but it correlates well to direct measurements and is, therefore, a good indicator of body fat percentage.

For adults, BMI is calculated using the following formula:
$$\text{weight (lb)} \div [\text{height (in)}^2] \times 703$$

Example: weight = 150 lbs; height = 5'5" (65")
Calculation: $[150 \div (65)^2] \times 703 = 24.96$ OR:
$150 \div (65 \times 65) \times 703 = 24.96$ OR:
$150 \div 4225 \times 703 = 24.96$

If you'd like to avoid doing the math yourself, you can use an on-line BMI calculator (such as the one available at my own Web site [www.sasseguide.com]), which performs the calculation for you, or you can use a BMI chart (see chart on following page).

A BMI chart is a simplified way to determine your BMI. Simply find your height on the vertical chart, and then move horizontally until you find the column that expresses your weight.

Chart source: Ethicon Endo-Surgery, Inc., Allergan, Inc. and EndoGastric Solutions, Inc.

	Height (ft)									
Weight (lbs)	4'9"	4'11"	5'1"	5'3"	5'5"	5'7"	5'9"	5'11"	6'1"	6'3"
154	33	31	29	27	26	24	23	22	20	19
165	36	33	31	29	28	26	24	23	22	21
176	38	36	33	31	29	28	26	25	23	22
187	40	38	35	33	31	29	28	26	25	24
198	43	40	37	35	33	31	29	28	26	25
209	45	42	40	37	35	33	31	29	28	26
220	48	44	42	39	37	35	33	31	29	28
231	50	47	44	41	39	36	34	32	31	29
243	52	49	46	43	40	38	36	34	32	30
254	55	51	48	45	42	40	38	35	34	32
265	57	53	50	47	44	42	39	37	35	33
276	59	56	52	49	46	43	41	39	37	35
287	62	58	54	51	48	45	42	40	38	36
298	64	60	56	53	50	47	44	42	39	37
309	67	62	58	55	51	48	46	43	41	39
320	69	64	60	57	53	50	47	45	42	40
331	71	67	62	59	55	52	49	46	44	42
342	74	69	65	61	57	54	51	48	45	43
353	76	71	67	63	59	55	52	49	47	44
364	78	73	69	64	61	57	54	51	48	46
375	81	76	71	66	62	59	56	52	50	47
386	83	78	73	68	64	61	57	54	51	48
397	86	80	75	70	66	62	59	56	53	50
408	88	82	77	72	68	64	60	57	54	51
419	90	84	79	74	70	66	62	59	56	53
430	93	87	81	76	72	67	64	60	57	54
441	95	89	83	78	73	69	65	62	59	55
452	98	91	85	80	75	71	67	63	60	57
463	100	93	87	82	77	73	69	65	61	58

Weight Category	BMI
Normal Weight	19–24.9
Overweight	25–29.9
Obese	30–39.9
Morbidly Obese	40–Greater

APPENDIX C: EXERCISES YOU CAN DO AT HOME

You don't have to join a fancy health club or gym to exercise. There are hundreds of ways to exercise right in your own home. Here are some ideas on specific exercises you might want to try. Consult a qualified sports trainer or other such professional for full instructions and guidance on performing any exercise mentioned here in a safe and effective manner. Consult your physician before undertaking any exercise activity or regimen.

EXERCISE	EXPLANATION
Air Chair	Sit against a wall and pretend you're sitting in a chair, thighs parallel to floor, arms out straight.
All Fours Bottoms Up Walk	Get on your hands and feet with your butt up in air, then "walk" on all fours.
Arches	Lie on your back and arch your hips off the floor while letting only your feet and the crown of your head touch the floor. Then slowly lean to your left and then to your right to test your balance. OR, from the arch position, quickly flip over so you're facing down. Repeat.
Backward Run or Sprint	Find a clear, safe path and run or sprint backward.
Bear Crawl	On hands and feet, go forward or backward. Don't just shuffle your legs; try to bring each foot far forward for each step. Try to keep your shins parallel to the floor; not angled up high.
Bend Over and Reach Back	Squat deeply and reach back between your feet as far as possible.
Box Jumps	Stand in front of a sturdy weight bench, wide stool, or chair. Then jump up, down, up, etc. Let your legs bend when you lands so you land to absorb the shock and to avoid jolting avoid jolting your knees. You can also jump sideways.

Break Dance	Get on your hands and toes and quickly hop from toe to toe. Then flip around so that you're facing upward while your hands and feet remain on the ground.
Broad Jumps or Triple Jumps	From a standing position, jump forward as far as possible. Or, begin with the standing broad jump; then, upon landing on your right leg, quickly hop forward to the left leg and land on both feet.
Calf Jump	Jump as high as possible using only the calf muscles; keep knees slightly bent.
Car Pushes or Pulls	Push or pull a car on a flat surface (make sure someone else is at the brake!). Do with or without a harness. Or, use another heavy object to push it, pull it, go sideways or at 45 degree angles.
Carry; Squat; Press	Carry a heavy object for a specified distance, then do squats or lunges, then overhead press.
Chop or Dig	Use a yard tool, such as shovel, to dig or carry dirt or rock for a distance. Or use a sledge-hammer to chop overhead or sideways repeatedly for a time or for a number of repetitions.
Crab Walk	Sit on the floor, then use your hands to raise your butt of the ground. Using your hands and feet, "walk" forward, backward, and sideways.
Crocodile Roll	Lie on your back, arms tight to your sides and feet together. Lift your legs off the floor and begin rolling left, right, etc., without letting your legs touch the floor.
Cross-County Skier	Mimic cross-country skiing, using arms and legs.
Crunch Up or Candle	Lie on your back, legs straight up vertically, then lift your butt off the ground.
Crunches	Do regular crunches, twist your torso as you come up each time, or do crunches on an incline.

Deep Push-up with Reverse	Starting in a normal push-up position, dip your head down and glide your torso forward until the hips are dipped down to the floor. Reverse the movements.
Dip	Facing away from a sturdy bench, chair, or stool, squat down. Plant your hands on the bench behind you and extend your legs out in front of you. Use your arms to push yourself up and slowly lower yourself.
Dive Bomber	From a standing position, fall forward into a push-up position. Do a push-up, then stand back up.
Duck Walk	Hands on your hips or behind your head, squat halfway down, and walk forward, backward, and sideways. walk forward, to sides, back.
Dumbbells	Lots of options! Use dumbbells to do chest presses; curls; tricep overhead extensions; lying tricep extensions; overhead presses; squats, lunges, and punches and kicks (see Shadowboxing).
Flutter Kick	Lie on your back with your hands under your butt. Raise your legs slightly and flutter them up and down.
Forward Rolls	Start in a standing position or a jog, then drop into a somersault roll, get up, and roll again.
Hand and Leg Opposites	Kneel on all fours, then slowly raise your right arm and left leg outward so they're parallel to the floor. Hold briefly, then alternate with the opposite arm and leg. You can remain in one spot or crawl across the floor. Or, do this while lying face down on the floor or on a stability ball.
Handstand	Get into a butt-up-high push-up position, then snap legs up fast like getting into a handstand, if you get tired then do push-ups.
High Knees	March in place with high knees, arms out straight ahead.

Inchworm	Stand like you're touching toes, then slowly finger your hands out as far as possible. Shuffle your feet toward your hands. Repeat.
Iron Cross	Lie on your back on a mat, with your arms out to your sides. Keeping your shoulders flat on the mat, swing foot to opposite hand. Repeat, alternating feet each time.
Jump and Sprint	Do a running or standing long jump. Upon landing, run or sprint.
Jump Rope	Keep you knees slightly bent to avoid jarring.
Jumping Butt Kicker	Begin in a standing position, then jump as high as possible while kicking (your own) butt.
Jumping Jacks	Do a standard jumping jack or vary it with one leg to the front and the other to the rear.
Kneeling Inchworm	Get into a kneeling push-up position. Walk your fingers out in front of you as far as possible, then walk them back to your starting position.
Kneeling to Hop	Kneel, then hop up into a standing position.
Leg Circles	Stand and lift one foot off the ground while keeping the leg straight. Then move the leg in small-to-big circles in front of you, behind you, and to the side of you. Or kneel, lift one leg, and make circles from that position.
Leg Lifts	To work the muscles in the back of your legs), kneel on a mat and place your elbows and forearms on the mat. Balance on one knee so that your back is parallel to the mat, raise the other leg in the air so that your thigh is parallel to the mat, and bend it at the knee. Place a small ball or bag behind that knee. Slowly raise and lower the leg without dropping the ball or bag. Repeat several times, then switch to the other leg. To work the muscles in the front of your thighs, sit with both legs straight in front of you. Lift one foot up about six inches, making sure your foot is flexed. Repeat several times, then switch to the other leg.

Leg Side Raise	Lie on your on side and support your head, then then slowly lift and lower one leg, keeping your toes pointed forward (not upward). Repeat several times, then switch to the other leg.
Leg Spread	Lying on your back with your hands under your bottom, slowly lift your legs, spread them, bring them back together, and lower your legs, being careful not to let them touch the ground. Repeat several times.
Leg Swing	Begin by sitting upright on the floor with your legs flat in front of you. Then lift your legs off the floor and swing them left, right, etc. Your arms may swing in the opposite direction to maintain balance.
Leg Clock Squat Down	Start with your left foot off a mat, hands on hips. As you squat, bring your left toe to a 12:00 position without touching the mat. Then return to your staring position. Then squat and go to 1:00. Repeat to 6:00, then switch legs.
Leg Hop	Using one or both legs at a time, hop forward, backward, to the side, and so forth.
Leg Squat or Jump Squat	Perform squats while standing on one or both legs. Or, you can squat and step forward, sideways, or backward down a line. Or you can squat and then jump up for more explosiveness.
Lunge	You can lunge forward, back, or to the side. For extra resistance, do lunges while holding dumbbells.
Lunge and Bend Over	Lunge forward, then bend over and reach your arms around your forward leg.
Medicine Ball	Hold a medicine ball while doing curls, squats, lunges, crunches, leg lifts, and other exercises. Throw the ball back and forth with a partner. Do push-ups with your hands placed on the ball.

Mogul Jump	With legs pressed together and knees slightly bent, quickly hop from side to side (mimicking a skier jumping over moguls).
Mountain Climber	Get into a push-up position, then alternate your feet as though you're running in place.
Monkey Walk	Squat down on a mat and place both fists on the mat. Keeping your torso upright, "walk," one step at a time, across the room. Stand up and jog back to the mat. Repeat.
Prone Cobras	Lying face down, arch upward to bring your legs, arms, and head back as far as possible.
Prone or Side Iso-Abs (Planks)	Lying face down, push up to lift your bodyweight onto your toes and forearms, then slowly lower yourself back down. To make the exercise more challenging, do this while keeping one leg raised. Rotate to your side, then down. To do a "reverse plank," lie on your back and sit up so that your forearms are supporting your upper body, then lift your bottom off the floor. Slowly lower it, being careful not to let it touch the mat, and lift it again.
Push-ups	You can do all kinds of push-ups: close, wide, regular, on a decline, with a clap, on your knees, against a wall (easier), or while pushing against a stability ball or medicine ball. Try working some safe variations into your movements!
Resistance Band Punch or Press	Bands can be affixed to a wall with an eye bolt and snap link or simply looped around a fixed object. Face away from the band's anchor point and grasp the handles, then step one leg forward as you simultaneously punch with the hand on the same side.
Resistance Band Rotation	Start be either standing or kneeling. Face away from the anchor point, point, grab a handle with each hand and bring them together over your head, then bend forward and twist.

Resistance Band Rows	Face a wall and grasp the band handles, then step one leg forward. Pull both bands simultaneously or alternate between bands.
Resistance Band Swimmer	Face the band's anchor point, pull the handles downward beside your hips, then bend forward slightly or do reverse swimmers.
Resistance Band—Other Things	Stand on the middle anchor point and do curls or front or side raises.
Roller Coaster	Lie face down and lower your body as if you're going under a low fence, straighten arms, arch back, sink hips, get up, then reverse back to start position.
Rope Exercises	Sling a rope or belt over a sturdy overhead bar or other object (tree branch, beam, etc.). Facing the bar, grasp the ends of the rope or belt and lean back to do incline pullups. The farther you lean back, the harder it will be. Or, face away from the bar and lean forward to do chest presses. The lower or more horizontal you are to the ground, the more difficult it will be. Or, face the bar and lean back while keeping your elbows stationary in front of you to do curls. Or, face away from the bar and keep your elbows stationary over your head to work triceps. Or, face away from the bar, extend your arms out sideways and then bring your extended arms together for "pec dec." Or, face the bar and lean back and raise yourself by extending your arms straight out to your sides to work your rear deltoids. Or, place a few knots in the rope and climb it. Or, do single-arm decline pulls.
Running in Place	This is a great exercise to do while you're watching TV.
Shadowboxing and Kicking	Pretend you're facing an opponent and then box and kick. Try doing this with a dumbbell in each hand or with a second person with hand mitts (and no dumbbell!). Do punches, hooks, upper-cuts, knees, elbows, kicks, etc. A good combo is left punch, right punch, left hook, right hook,

left uppercut, right uppercut, repeat. Or, do a front kick, advance forward, then punch and mix it up.

Shrimp	Lie on your side, arch into a half-moon-shaped curve, and push both feet straight out, causing your hips and bottom to shoot back, as you reach your hands toward your feet. Flip to the other side and repeat.
Shoulder Shrugs	Holding a dumbbell in each hand, shrug your shoulders up and down.
Shuffle Side to Side	Shuffle your feet quickly to move yourself while keeping your upper body upright. You may also cross your feet as you shuffle them and twist your upper body as your feet cross.
Ski and Lean	From a standing position, squat down. Shift your weight so that 80 percent of it is on your left leg. Then shift your weight to the other leg.
Skip Up	This is merely exaggerated skipping. Bring one knee up high, then hop. Bring the other knee up, then hop. Repeat.
Sit-ups	See Crunches.
Spider Crawl	Face down with your hands and feet on floor and limbs extended about 45 degrees out to each corresponding side. Then swing your limbs to crawl along while keeping limbs extended.
Sprawl	Begin in a standing position, then shoot the legs back (like a wrestler avoiding a leg takedown), drop, and get back up.
Squat-Thrust-Jumps	Squat down, do a push-up, then jump up or do a pull-up.
Stability Ball	Use a stability ball to do push-ups or to sit or lie on as you do curls, leg lifts, chest stretches, sit-ups, and other exercises.

Stability Ball Arm Extensions

Get into a push-up position with your forearms on the ball, then extend your arms forward to your elbows, then roll ball back to your wrist area, repeat. You can do this while kneeling, as well.

Stability Ball Bridge and Leg Curl

Lie on your back with your heels on the ball, then bridge by lifting your hips and bottom off the floor so that your torso is straight, then use your feet to roll the ball under your bottom.

Stability Ball Hand and Leg Opposites

Lie face down with the ball under your stomach or sternum, then slowly raise your right arm and left leg outward so they are parallel to the floor. Hold briefly, then alternate with the opposite arm and leg.

Stability Ball Hyperextension

Lie face down with the ball under your stomach and hands on your head. Bend forward toward the floor and then arch upward.

Stability Ball Leg Raise Crunch

Sit on the ball, lean back slightly, and alternate bringing each knee to your chest.

Stability Ball Leg Jackknife

Lie face up with your legs straight in front of you and your toes resting on the ball. Using your hands, push your body up so that it is parallel to the floor. Using your feet, roll the ball forward and back as far as possible.

Stability Ball Pec Dec (2 balls)

Lie face down with your forearms clinched tightly to your chest and a ball resting under each forearm. Spread your arms outward away from your chest, keeping your arms bent at 90-degree angles.

Stability Ball Pelvic Raise

Lie on your back with the ball under your calves, then raise your hips and bottom so that your torso is in line with your calves.

Stability Ball Pike

Get into a push-up position with the ball under your shins, then roll the ball forward and lift up your bottom.

Stability Ball Reverse Hyperextension

Lie face down so that your stomach is on the ball. Lean forward so your weight is on your forearms, then pull your legs upward off the floor until your body and legs are in a straight line.

Stability Ball Roller Coaster — Kneel down and place the ball under your chest, then push forward with your feet so that you roll forward toward your head. Use your hands to stop your movement and to push yourself back to the starting position.

Stability Ball Single Leg Lateral — Stand with the ball about three feet to your side. Extend the adjacent leg and rest your foot on the ball, then roll the ball forward and back with your foot.

Stability Ball Wall Rollout — Stand facing a wall while pushing the ball against the wall at eye level, then lean forward as you roll the ball extended above your head, then down.

Stability Ball Wall Squat — Stand with your your back about two feet away from a wall and place the ball against your lower back area. Then lean back against the ball and slowly squatdown and raise back up.

Stability Ball Twists — Get into a push-up position with the ball under your knees or thighs, then rotate your hips to the left and the right.

Step Ups — Step on and off a bench, stool, chair, stair, or other such object. As you step up, bring the other foot up so that you are standing on both feet. Step down, then bring the other foot down.

Supine Bicycle — Lie on your back, and move as though you are pedaling a bike. As the left knee comes toward you, bring your right elbow to it, and so forth.

Lying Leg Kick to Standing — Sit upright as though you've been knocked on the ground while standing and an advancing opponent is approaching you. Sit on your right hip and right elbow or hand as your right leg kicks, while your left foot plants on the floor to move. Also practice standing up from this position by swinging your right leg back under your pelvis.

Swimmer	Lying face down with your head up high, mimic swimming by paddling your extended arms and legs up and down.
Teeter Totter and Stretch	Sit with your legs flat on the floor. Lift your legs up and roll backward until your feet touch the floor above your head. Then go to your starting position and touch your toes.
Toe Hops	From a standing position, make quick hops on your toes. Concentrate on using only your calf muscles.
Toe Raises	Stand on the edge of a step or curb with only your toes on the floor or ground (hold onto a stationary object for support). Using your calf muscles, raise your toes up and down.
Tuck Jump	Jump high while bringing your knees to your chest.
Wall Walk	Lie on your back with your bottom touching a wall and your legs raised and resting on the wall, then "walk" your feet up the wall as you lift your bottom off the floor. "Walk" back down.
Wishbone Kicks	Lie on your back with your feet together and pushing on a wall, your legs bent 90 degrees. Use one leg to push your bottom away from the wall. As you're doing this, straighten the other leg and point it upward. Repeat, alternating legs.
180-Degree Leaps	Stand on one foot, then leap and twist around 180 degrees and land on your opposite foot. Hold your position for three seconds, then leap to your starting position. Repeat, alternating legs.
Two-Person Face Off	Stand about 10 yards away from a partner. As each person advances toward the other, one tries to tag or tackle his or her partner as the other tries to avoid being tagged or tackled.
Two-Person Foot Throws	One person lies on his or her back with knees bent and at the chest; the other person stands about five feet in front of his or her partner's feet

and gently tosses a ball (or a stability or medicine ball) to the other person's feet. The person lying down catches the ball, then throws it back, with his or her feet.

Two-Person Leg Lift and Push	One person lies on on his or her back with with legs extended straight up vertically while the second person grasps the lying person's feet and pulls his or her legs downward toward the floor. The lying person tries to prevent his or her feet from landing on the floor by returning his/her legs to the start position
Two-Person Push-ups	One person either kneels on all fours or gets into a "bottom up" position, with only his or her hands and toes touching the floor. The other person places his or her hands on the first person's back and does push-ups.
Two-Person Medicine Ball Soccer	Play soccer using a medicine ball.
Two-Person Medicine Ball Toss	Toss a medicine ball back and forth. You can add lunges, twists, squats, and other exercise movements.
Two-Person Medicine Ball Pick-up	Stand side by side, about three feet apart. One person holds a medicine ball. Both people squat, and the medicine ball is placed on the ground between the two people. The other person picks up the ball, then both people stand up. Repeat.
Two-Person Rows	One person lies on the ground. The second person stands over the lying person with his or her feet planted at the person's waist area. Then the standing person grasps graps the other's hands and slowly pulls his or her upper body off the floor.
Two-Person "Sumo Wrestling"	Two people face off in a marked area with soft ground and attempt to remove the other person from the area.

APPENDIX D: MOVING IN THE RIGHT DIRECTION
Provided by iMetabolic

Walking is a low-cost, safe fitness activity that almost everyone can do. Increasing physical activity will help you work better, sleep better, feel better, and look better. It's important to make intentional physical activity a part of your daily life while you are losing weight, and it's essential to maintaining weight loss.

Did you know that the average American walks between 3,000 and 5,000 steps a day?

We all have to start somewhere. Make it a point to move more any way you can. Look at extra steps as an opportunity to burn more calories. It is critical to make activity a part of your lifestyle while you are losing weight because activity will be absolutely essential when it comes to maintaining that weight loss.

STEP LOG

At the end of the day, record the steps from your pedometer on the log. At the end of each week, add up the number of total steps you took that week. Divide the total by the number of days you recorded for the average. Your goal is to increase your daily average every week by 500 steps or or by 10 percent (whichever is greater).

	Week of ___	Week of ___	Week of ___	Week of ___
Monday				
Tuesday				
Wednesday				
Thursday				
Friday				
Saturday				
Sunday				
TOTAL				
AVERAGE				

	Week of ___	Week of ___	Week of ___	Week of ___
Monday				
Tuesday				
Wednesday				
Thursday				
Friday				
Saturday				
Sunday				
TOTAL				
AVERAGE				

Appendix E: Sources Of Protein

The following table shows a breakdown of calories from protein and fat, as well as the total number of calories, in various foods. It's important to choose foods that are high in protein, low in fat, and low in carbs so that you can get the maximum amount of protein in your diet while you're creating a calorie deficit (cutting calories). By doing so, you help to ensure that you retain your lean body mass.

FOOD	PORTION	CALORIES	PROTEIN GRAMS	FAT GRAMS
Almonds, roasted	1/4 cup	210	8	19
Beans, baked, vegetarian	1/2 cup	130	6	0
Beans, refried, non-fat	1/2 cup	130	8	0
Black beans, cooked	1/2 cup	115	8	0
Boca® Burger	1 patty	150	15	5
Buttermilk, low-fat	1/2 cup	55	5	1
Canadian bacon	2 slices	85	11	4
Cheese, low-fat	1 oz.	50	7	2
Chicken breast, skinless, baked or grilled	3 oz.	140	27	3
Chicken thigh, skinless, baked or grilled	1 thigh	110	13	6
Chicken, canned with broth	1/2 can (2.5 oz)	75	16	1
Chicken, deli lunchmeat	2 oz.	60	12	1
Chickpeas, cooked	1/2 cup	100	6	1
Clams, cooked	10 small	90	14	1
Cod, baked or grilled	3 oz.	90	19	1

FOOD	PORTION	CALORIES	PROTEIN GRAMS	FAT GRAMS
Cottage cheese, low-fat 1%	1/2 cup	80	14	1
Crab, canned	3 oz.	85	17	1
Egg subsitute, liquid	1/4 cup	55	8	2
Egg, large, cooked without fat	1	70	6	5
Gardenburger®	1 patty	120	14	4
Great Northern beans	1/2 cup	70	6	0
Ground beef, lean, broiled	3 oz.	185	22	10
Halibut, baked or grilled	3 oz.	120	23	3
Kidney beans	1/2 cup	100	7	0
Lentils, cooked	1/2 cup	115	9	0
Lima beans, cooked	1/2 cup	115	7	0
Lobster	3 oz.	80	17	1
Meatloaf	3 oz.	180	14	11
Milk, non-fat	1/2 cup	40	4	0
Morningstar Farms® meatless breakfast patty	1 patty	80	10	3
Navy beans, cooked	1/2 cup	150	10	1
Orange roughy, baked or grilled	3 oz.	90	18	1
Oysters, canned	3 oz.	60	6	2
Peanut butter, reduced-fat	2 tbsp.	190	8	12

FOOD	PORTION	CALORIES	PROTEIN GRAMS	FAT GRAMS
Pinto beans, cooked	1/2 cup	110	7	1
Quaker® Weight Control Oatmeal	1 packet	160	7	3
Ricotta cheese, low-fat	1/4 cup	60	7	3
Salmon, baked or grilled	3 oz.	195	22	11
Salmon, canned pink	3 oz.	125	16	7
Scallops, cooked	2 large	45	9	0
Sea bass, baked or grilled	3 oz.	105	20	2
Shrimp, cooked	4 medium	85	11	1
Snapper, baked or grilled	3 oz.	110	22	1
Soybeans (edamame), cooked	1/2 cup	100	10	3
Soy milk	1/2 cup	65	5	2
Split peas, cooked	1/2 cup	115	8	0
Tilapia, baked or grilled	3 oz.	110	22	2
Tofu, soft	1/2 cup	75	8	5
Tuna, canned, packed in water	1/2 can (2.5 oz)	90	19	0
Turkey bologna	2 slices	140	8	12
Turkey breast, skinless	3 oz.	75	17	1
Turkey, ground, cooked	3 oz.	180	21	11
Yogurt, low-fat, unsweetened	6 oz.	90	6	0

APPENDIX F: SPECIFIC DANGERS OF WEIGHT GAIN AND OBESITY

The human race has made several advancements over a period of time. Due to all these advancements life has become extremely sedentary. People don't do enough physical activity as a result more and more people are becoming victims of obesity.

Many people just don't bother to take their weight problems seriously. They feel it is just a cosmetic disorder. This is far from the truth. Obesity is a serious health problem and it causes around 300,000 deaths per year, second only to smoking.

Obesity leads to serious health problems which number north of thirty. The more notable health concerns are heart disease, high blood pressure, stroke, cancer, diabetes, osteoarthritis, gallstones, gallbladder disease, gout, and breathing problems like asthma. Thus, a person who is 40% overweight is said to be twice as likely to die prematurely as compared to an average weight person.

A short list of the different health problems caused by obesity includes:

Heart Disease & Stroke

A heart disease affects the normal functioning of the heart and it results in blood not circulating properly. Heart diseases can lead to problems like a heart attack, congestive heart failure, sudden cardiac death, angina (chest pain), or abnormal heart rhythm. When a person suffers from stroke it results in blood and oxygen not reaching the brain.

High levels of cholesterol and triglycerides (blood fats) in the blood can lead to strokes and heart disease. Doctors say that even a weight gain of 20 pounds doubles the risk of heart disease.

Type 2 Diabetes

In type 2 diabetes the blood sugar of the person goes above the normal level. When a person is obese or overweight it affects the cells causing them to become less effective in removing sugar from blood. As a result there is more pressure put on the insulin producing cells as a result of which they gradually stop working.

Weight gain increases the risk of developing type 2 diabetes and it has been found that 80% of the people suffering from diabetes are overweight or obese.

Cancer

Cancer is a leading cause of death in the U.S. Though cancer need not necessarily originate from obesity but obesity does increase the chances of certain types of cancers. These cancers include cancers of the colon, esophagus, and kidney, and uterine and postmenopausal breast cancer in women.

It is believed that being overweight or obese causes the fat cells in the body to make hormones that affect cell growth and can lead to cancer.

Liver Disease

When fat builds up in the liver it can lead to liver disease and can result in injury and inflammation in the liver. Fat can also cause severe liver damage, cirrhosis and even liver failure.

High Blood Pressure

Being overweight or obese is a leading cause of high blood pressure. According to doctors being 20% overweight makes you eight times more likely to suffer from high blood pressure as compared to an averaged weight person.

Sleep Apnea

When a person stops breathing for short periods in the night, the condition is termed as sleep apnea. Sleep apnea is caused when fat gets stored around the neck resulting in narrowing of the airway. Fat stored in the body can also cause inflammation in the neck, this can also causes sleep apnea.

Gout

Gout is caused due to a high level of uric acid in the blood. Sometimes uric acid forms into solid stone or crystal masses that get deposited in the joints. Gout is a problem that is usually experienced by overweight people.

Problems in Women

Women who are obese often suffer from irregularities in the menstrual cycles and infertility. If a woman is obese during pregnancy it increases the risk of death of both the mother and the child. It also leads to an increase the risk of maternal high blood pressure by 10 times. Obesity during pregnancy can also cause birth defects, particularly neural tube defects.

Gallstones

Being overweight is a major factor for the formation of gallstones. Gallstones are solid clusters that form in the gallbladder. They are usually made of cholesterol and overweight people produce more cholesterol, hence they are at risk.

Urinary Stress Incontinence

A large, heavy abdomen and relaxation of the pelvic muscles, especially associated with the effects of childbirth, may cause the valve on the urinary bladder to be weakened, leading to leakage of urine with coughing, sneezing, or laughing.

A healthy diet and regular physical activity are both important for maintaining a healthy weight. Even a small decrease in calories consumed and an increase in physical activity can help prevent weight gain or facilitate weight loss.

Hyperlipidemia

Hyperlipidemia refers to high cholesterol in the body and it is caused by a build up of fatty substances in the arteries. Due to this the arteries narrow and become hard as a result of which blood flow to the heart goes down.

This can result in chest pain and heart attacks. Hyperlipidemia is caused by several factors but an increase in weight is a leading cause.

Osteoarthritis

Osteoarthritis is a join disorder where the joint bone cartilage wears away. It usually affects the knees, hips, and lower back. Osteoarthritis is usually caused by an increase in the body weight as it exerts extra pressure on the joints and cartilage. People who have more body fat also face the risk of inflammation at the joints and this may cause osteoarthritis. There is an 8 to 12% increase in the risk of developing Osteoarthritis with every two pound increase in weight.

Varicose Veins

Varicose veins are formed when valves in the veins weaken and due to this veins permanently dilate. Blood is not pumped around the body instead it pools in the veins. Having excess weight in the body leads to varicose veins and when a person looses weight it helps in the treatment.

Psychological and Social Effects

Probably the psychological and social effects of obesity are the most painful. When a person suffers from obesity he often looses confidence and feels unattractive. Obese people are often made fun of and discriminated as a result of which they find it really hard to lead a happy life, many start suffering from depression.

Need to Loose Weight

These dangers of obesity make it extremely important to loose weight. But here again there is another problem. People often try to loose weight quickly with the help of fad diets. But it must be remembered that successful and happy weight loss takes time and one needs to be patient. Fad diets might help in loosing weight but they bring about weight loss by depriving the body of some necessary nutrients. This might cause further health complications.

The only healthy way to lose weight is by following a proper weight loss program that includes exercise and a reduced calorie diet. You should not aim too high in the beginning, you need to set attainable goals. Being patient is the key.

APPENDIX G: RISK FACTORS
AND RISK REDUCTION
AN INTERVIEW WITH MICHAEL J. BLOCK, MD

Michael J. Block, MD, is a colleague of mine. He's a national expert in cardiovascular disease, an associate professor at the University of Nevada School of Medicine, the founder and medical director of Saint Mary's Risk-Reduction Center, and the codirector of Saint Mary's Vascular Institute. I had a chance to talk with him about some of the risk factors caused by being overweight or obese—and some risk-reduction factors.

KS: What is meant by the term "risk reduction"?

MB: We all pay great lip service to the concept of preventative health, but it is very clear that, in our personal lives and medical interactions, many of us focus on acute medical issues rather than on long-term preventative measures. We actually have tremendous ability to determine an individual's personal risk of developing heart disease, stroke, and other chronic medical conditions, and we have multiple tools, both through lifestyle changes and medications, to reduce this risk dramatically. We just need a better system for getting people to focus on their individual risk and to take appropriate steps to reduce it.

KS: What is the major risk to long-term health as you see it?

MB: In a word: atherosclerosis. Taken together, heart disease and stroke are the number one cause of death in the United States and, perhaps more important as our population ages, they are tremendously expensive and are a major cause of hospitalization, loss of independence, and diminished quality of life. The primary cause of heart disease and stroke is atherosclerosis, a buildup of cholesterol plaque in the blood vessels that bring oxygen and nutrients to the heart, brain, and other organs. To a great extent, atherosclerosis and its complications are preventable. Major controllable risk factors for atherosclerosis include high blood pressure, unfavorable cholesterol, high blood sugar, smoking, and other related factors.

KS: How do those risks diminish in people who lose weight?

MB: Most risk factors for heart disease and stroke, including blood pressure, cholesterol, and elevated blood sugar (diabetes and pre-diabetes), are closely associated with being overweight or obese. Unfortunately, in our society we tend to focus on treating these conditions with medications; however, aggressive lifestyle interventions, including weight loss and increased physical activity, can also be effective. People who successfully maintain weight loss can often be treated with significantly less medication. Even small reductions in weight, as little as five to ten pounds, if maintained, can have significant beneficial effects on these risk factors. From a public health perspective, I also believe that we need to begin to focus on the concept of primordial prevention, which is the prevention of these risk factors in the first place through maintenance of healthy weight and better diet and exercise habits.

KS: What's the hardest thing for people to do to persevere and stick with a weight-loss program?

MB: I think it is hard for people to recognize that even small changes, if maintained over time, can have dramatic health benefits. As I always remind my patients, it does no good to lose substantial amounts of weight over a couple of months if you are just going to regain that weight the next month. Many of my patients have lost and regained hundreds of pounds over their lifetimes. How long an individual can maintain that weight loss is really the key. Remember that losing two pounds each and every month, which doesn't sound like a lot, adds up to 25 pounds in a year and 50 pounds in two years. Now, most people don't need to lose that much weight to experience positive effects on their health and quality of life. In the federally funded Diabetes Prevention Program, weight loss of about 7 percent of total body weight, maintained over a few years, decreased the risk of developing diabetes by about 65 percent. We need to stop thinking about "diets," which tend to focus on short-term results, and start thinking about long-term lifestyle change.

KS: How do you specifically encourage your patients to maintain their efforts to reduce risk and live healthier lives?

MB: Most health care providers have a tendency to focus on numbers—weight, waist circumference, BMI, blood pressure, cholesterol, blood sugar, and the like. These things are certainly important, but they are somewhat abstract for many people and they are not always as motivating as they could be. While I certainly do encourage people to "know their numbers," I think it's important to put them into the context of what it means for their quality of life. I try to focus on the relationship between these numbers and the reduction of risk of heart failure, stroke, and other quality-of-life-robbing cardiovascular events. I also remind patients about how much better they feel and how much more they can do in their everyday lives at a healthier weight and with better dietary and exercise habits.

KS: Any other thoughts on the medical impact of obesity and on the health impact of life-changing weight-loss programs like the iMetabolic program?

MB: As a cardiovascular specialist, I am always struck by the lack of progress we have seen in heart disease and stroke prevention over the past decades. We have tremendous new technologies for treating heart disease and stroke when they occur but, obviously, prevention is the best intervention. Over the last few decades we have done a better job of lowering blood pressure, improving cholesterol, and getting people to quit smoking, yet we have seen little change in the overall incidence of heart attack and stroke. This is because the downside of the epidemics of obesity, diabetes, and metabolic syndrome have overwhelmed the upside that we have seen in these more traditional risk factors. In an environment like ours that is essentially toxic to the blood vessels, people need individualized tools like the iMetabolic program to assist them in maintaining more heart-healthy lifestyle habits and improving their quality of life.

KS: Thank you very much Dr. Bloch. We all appreciate the work you are doing in risk reduction for cardiovascular disease.

Michael J. Bloch, M.D.
Associate Professor, University of Nevada School of Medicine
Founder and Medical Director, Saint Mary's Risk Reduction Center
Co-Director, Saint Mary's Vascular Institute
Reno, NV
www.saintmarysreno.org

References

Articles

Blue, L. Obesity is contagious. *Time*: In partnership with CNN. July 25, 2007.

How many calories have you burned? (2007). *USA Today*/Lifestyle.

Jacobson, M.F. (2005) Liquid Candy: How soft drinks are harming Americans' Health. Center for Science in the Public Interest.

Lambert, C. (2004). The way we eat now. *Harvard Magazine*.

Martin, A. (2007). Makers of sodas try a new pitch: They are healthy. *New York Times*.

Martin, D.S. If you see it, you will eat it, experts say. CNN.com

McGregor, W. Using portion size to cut calories.

Sklar, B. (2007). Get the candy jar out of your office. *That's Fit*.

Surprising reasons why we overeat. (2007). WNBC.com/Health

Vangsness, S. (2005). Mastering the Mindful Meal. Brigham and Women's Hospital (teaching affiliate of Harvard Medical School).

Warner, J. (2005). Six secrets of successful weight loss. WebMD Health.

Books

100 Must-Read Life-Changing Books (Bloomsbury Good Reading Guides)
by Nick Rennison (editor)

All We Have Is All We Need: Daily Steps Toward a Peaceful Life
by Karen Casey.

The Art of Changing: Your Path to a Better Life by Susan Peabody.

Being In Balance: 9 Principles for Creating Habits to Match Your Desires
by Wayne W. Dyer.

Believing in Myself: Self Esteem Daily Meditations by Ernie Larsen.

The Biology of Belief: Unleashing the Power of Consciousness, Matter,
& Miracles by Bruce H. Lipton Ph.D.

Change Your Mind And Your Life Will Follow: 12 Simple Principles
by Karen Casey.

Change Your Thoughts – Change Your Life: Living the Wisdom of the Tao
by Wayne W. Dyer.

Changing Your Course: The 5-Step Guide to Getting the Life You Want
(Live What You Love) by Robert Blanchard and Melinda Blanchard.

Choices: Taking Control of Your Life and Making It Matter by Melody Beattie.

Each Day a New Beginning: Daily Meditations for Women by Karen Casey.

Eating Mindfully 2003 by S. Albers.

Finding Your Own North Star: Claiming the Life You Were Meant to Live
by Martha Beck.

Life Changes: Using the Power of Change to Transform Your Life
by Jennifer Lewis-Hall.

REFERENCES

Living the Wisdom of the Tao: The Complete Tao Te Ching and Affirmations by Wayne W. Dyer.

Love Yourself, Heal Your Life Workbook (Insight Guide) by Louise Hay.

Mindful Eating 101 by S. Albers.

Mindless Eating: Why We Eat More Than We Think by Brian Wansink.

On The Shoulders Of Giants: 33 New Ways to Guide Yourself To Greatness by Rhondalynn Korolak.

Quiet Mind: One-Minute Retreats from a Busy World by David Kundtz.

The New Codependency: Help and Guidance for Today's Generation by Melody Beattie.

The Promise of a New Day: A Book of Daily Meditations (Hazelden Meditations) by Karen Casey and Martha Vanceburg.

The Secret by Rhonda Byrne.

This Is Not the Life I Ordered: 50 Ways to Keep Your Head Above Water When Life Keeps Dragging You Down by Deborah Collins Stephens, Michealene Cristini Risley, Jackie Speier, andJan Yanehiro (Author)

You Can Heal Your Life by Louise Hay.

Resources

Please note that this is only a partial list of resources and that it contains those that are most relevant and salient to this particular publication. A more robust list of health- and weight-loss-related resource information is available at www.sasseguide.com.

Bariatric Organizations

American Society of Bariatric Physicians (ASBP)
2821 South Parker Rd., Ste. 625, Aurora, CO 80014
303-770-2526   www.asbp.org
(The American Society of Bariatric Physicians is a leading national professional organization providing physicians and other health professionals with education in the medical management of weight loss and related medical conditions. Bariatric medicine is defined as the art and science of medical weight management and associated comorbidities.)

American Society for Metabolic & Bariatric Surgery
100 SW 75th St., Ste. 201, Gainesville, FL 32607
352-331-4900   www.asbs.org
(The purpose of the society is to advance the art and science of bariatric surgery by continued encouragement of its members to carry out the following mission: to improve the care and treatment of people with obesity and related diseases; to advance the science and understanding of metabolic surgery; to foster communication among health professionals in regard to obesity and related conditions; to be the recognized authority and

resource on metabolic and bariatric surgery; and to advocate for health care policy that ensures patient access to high-quality prevention and treatment of obesity.)

Diabetes Organizations

Joslin Diabetes Center
One Joslin Place, Boston, MA 02215
617-732-2400   www.joslin.org
(Joslin Diabetes Center is the only diabetes institution in the world that goes beyond a single focus. With efforts in these three critical areas, a synergy develops: researchers, clinicians, and educators collaborate in ways that produce cutting-edge scientific discovery, unique clinical care models, and pioneering educational strategies. This one-of-a-kind framework has an impact on people with diabetes locally, nationally, and across the globe.)

Juvenile Diabetes Research Foundation International
120 Wall St., New York, NY 10005-4001
800-533-2873   www.jdrf.org
(JDRF is the leader in research leading to a cure for type 1 diabetes in the world. It sets the global agenda for diabetes research, and it is the largest charitable foundation and advocate of diabetes science worldwide.)

National Diabetes Education Program
One Diabetes Way, Bethesda, MD 20814-9692
301-496-3583   www.ndep.nih.gov
(The National Diabetes Education Program is a federally funded program sponsored by the U.S. Department of Health and Human Services' National Institutes of Health and the Centers for Disease Control and Prevention. It includes more than 200 partners at the federal, state, and local levels that are working. together to improve the treatment and outcomes of people with diabetes, promote early diagnosis, and prevent or delay the onset of type 2 diabetes.)

State of Diabetes Complications in America
888-825-5249   www.stateofdiabetes.com
(This Web site is part of a national education program called the State of

Diabetes Complications in America, created by the American Association of Clinical Endocrinologists [AACE] in partnership with the members of the diabetes complications consortium, including the Amputee Coalition of America [ACA], Mended Hearts, National Federation of the Blind [NFB] and the National Kidney Foundation [NKF]. The consortium was formed to provide beneficial information to people with type 2 diabetes about how to reduce the risk of the health complications associated with the disease, as well as to provide support and encouragement to people who have experienced these serious health problems.)

Nutrition Organizations

American Society for Nutrition
9650 Rockville Pike, Bethesda, MD 20814
301-634-7050   www.nutrition.org
(The American Society for Nutrition [ASN] is a nonprofit organization dedicated to bringing together the world's top researchers, clinical nutritionists, and the world's industry to advance the knowledge and application of nutrition for the sake of humans and animals. Focus ranges from the most critical details of research and application to the broadest applications in society in the United States and around the world.)

National Agricultural Library Food and Nutrition Information Center
10301 Baltimore Ave., Beltsville, MD 20705-2351   www.nutrition.gov
(This organization's Web site is designed to provide users access to practical information on healthy eating, dietary supplements, fitness, and food safety information. The site is regularly updated with the latest news, and it features links to other interesting Web sites.)

Society for Nutrition Education (SNE)
9100 Purdue Rd., Ste. 200, Indianapolis, IN 46268
317-328-4627   www.sne.org
(SNE is dedicated to promoting effective nutrition education and communication to support and improve healthful behaviors. Its goal is to promote healthy communities through. nutrition education and advocacy.)

Obesity Organizations

North American Association for the Study of Obesity (NAASO)

The Obesity Society (AOA), 8630 Fenton St., Ste. 814, Silver Spring,
MD 20910 301-563-6526   www.obesity.org
(The Obesity Society is the leading scientific society dedicated to the study
of obesity. Since 1982, the Obesity Society has been committed to encouraging research on the causes and treatment of obesity and to keeping the
medical community and public informed of new advances.)

Women's Health Organizations

MGH Center for Women's Mental Health

Perinatal and Reproductive Psychiatry Program Simches Research Building
185 Cambridge St., Ste. 2200, Boston, MA 02114
617-724-7792   www.womensmentalhealth.org
(This organization's Web site provides a range of current information,
including discussion of new research findings in women's mental health
and the ways in which such investigations inform day-to-day clinical practice.
Despite the growing number of studies being conducted in women's health,
the clinical implications of such work are frequently controversial, leaving
patients with questions regarding the most appropriate path to follow.
The goal of this organization is to provide these resources to patients and
their doctors so that individual clinical decisions can be made in a thoughtful
and collaborative fashion.)

National Women's Health Resource Center

157 Broad St., Ste. 106, Red Bank, NJ 07701
800-986-9472   www.healthywomen.org
(This organization's Web site provides women in-depth, objective, physician-
approved information on a broad range of women's health issues.
With more than 100 topics in its health library, including the latest
medical advancements in each field, the site offers a robust level of
support for females.)

Sister to Sister: The Women's Heart Health Foundation
4701 Willard Ave., Ste.223, Chevy Chase, MD 20815
301-718-8033   www.sistertosister.org
(Sister to Sister is a 501(c)(3) nonprofit foundation dedicated to preventing
heart disease in women. The organization's goal is to promise women that
they have the power to protect their own hearts.)

Office on Women's Health
U.S. Department of Health & Human Services
800-994-9662   www.womenshealth.gov
(The Office on Women's Health [OWH] was established within the U.S.
Department of Health and Human Services. Its vision is to ensure that
"all women and girls are healthier and that they have a better sense of well-
being." Its mission is to "provide leadership and promote health equity
among women and girls through sex/gender-specific approaches.")

Women's Health Initiative (WHI)
2 Rockledge Ctr., Ste. 10018, MS 7936 6701, Rockledge Dr.,
Bethesda, MD 20892-7936
301-402-2900   www.nhlbi.nih.gov/whi
(The Women's Health Initiative [WHI] represents a major 15-year research
program to address the most common causes of death, disability and poor
quality of life in postmenopausal women–cardiovascular disease, cancer,
and osteoporosis.)

Women's Heart Foundation
P.O. Box 7827, West Trenton, NJ 08628
609-771-3778   www.womensheart.org
(Women's Heart Foundation is the "only non-governmental organization
that implements heart disease prevention projects." It consists of a coalition
of executive nurses, civic leaders, community health directors, hospitals,
women's heart centers, partners, providers, and corporate sponsors respond-
ing to the health crisis of women's heart disease and the urgent need for
prevention programs. WHF advocates for women and supports early
intervention and excellence of care of women.)

Government Organizations

Calorie Control Council
www.caloriecontrol.org
(This organization provides information on cutting calories and fat in one's diet, tips on achieving and maintaining a healthy weight, and understanding common low-calorie, reduced-fat foods and beverages (and the ingredients that make them possible.)

Food and Nutrition Service
United States Department of Agriculture Food & Nutrition Service
3101 Park Center Dr., Alexandria, VA 22302
www.fns.usda.gov/fns
(The Food and Nutrition Service [FNS], formerly known as the Food and Consumer Service, administers the nutrition assistance programs of the U.S. Department of Agriculture. One of their primary goals is to "improve the nation's nutrition and health")

Foundation for the National Institutes of Health
9650 Rockville Pike, Bethesda, MD 20814-3999
301-402-5311   www.fnih.org
(The Foundation for the National Institutes of Health was established by the United States Congress to support the mission of the National Institutes of Health [NIH]: to improve health through scientific discovery.)

National Institutes of Health
9000 Rockville Pike, Bethesda, MD 20892
301-496-4000   www.nih.gov
(The National Institutes of Health [NIH] is part of the U.S. Department of Health and Human Services, and it acts as the primary federal agency for conducting and supporting medical research. NIH scientists investigate ways to prevent disease as well as the causes, treatments, and even cures for common and rare diseases. Composed of 27 institutes and centers, the NIH provides leadership and financial support to researchers in every state and throughout the world.)

Office of the Surgeon General (OSG)

Department of Health & Human Services
Office of the Surgeon General
5600 Fishers Ln., Rm. 18-66, Rockville, MD 20857
301-443-4000   www.surgeongeneral.gov
(The surgeon general serves as America's chief health educator by providing Americans the best scientific information available on how to improve their health and reduce the risk of illness and injury. The surgeon general is appointed by the president of the United States with the advice and consent of the United States senate for a four-year term of office.)

National Weight Control Registry

Brown Medical School/The Miriam Hospital
Weight Control & Diabetes Research Center
196 Richmond St., Providence, RI 02903
800-606-6927   www.nwcr.ws
(Given the prevailing belief that few individuals succeed at long-term weight loss, the NWCR was founded to identify and investigate the characteristics of individuals who have succeeded at long-term weight loss. The NWCR is tracking over 5,000 individuals who have lost significant amounts of weight and kept it off for long periods.)

President's Council on Physical Fitness and Sports

Department of Health and Human Services
PCPFS, Department W, 200 Independence Ave., S.W., Rm. 738-H
Washington, D.C. 20201
202-690-9000   www.fitness.gov
(Site represents the health, physical activity, fitness and sports information Web site dedicated by the President's Council on physical fitness and sports.)

Weight-Control Information Network (WIN)

One WIN Wy., Bethesda, MD 20892-3665
877-946-4627   www.win.niddk.nih.gov
(WIN was established in 1994 to provide the general public, health professionals, the media, and the U.S. congress with up-to-date, science-based information on obesity, weight control, physical activity, and related nutritional issues.)

Web Sites: Obesity and Health

Aetna
www.intelihealth.com
(Aetna's mission is to empower people with trusted
solutions for healthier lives. This is accomplished by providing credible
information from the most trusted sources.)

eMedicineHealth
www.emedicinehealth.com
(Practical medical information on a wide range of topics is available at
this Web site. With more than 5,500 pages of health content, the site
contains articles written by physicians for patients and consumers.
eMedicineHealth also offers a RSS feeds to alert viewers on new and
updated content on the site.)

HealthCentral.com
www.healthcentral.com
(Another in a series of robust sites offering
content from Harvard Health Publications, A.D.A.M., HealthDay, and
Thompson's PDR. The site also has a newsletter and a robust portal of other
sites dedicated to obesity, nutrition, and other weight-related issues.)

MayoClinic.com
www.mayoclinic.com
(More than 3,300 physicians, scientists, and researchers
from Mayo Clinic share their expertise to empower you to manage your
health. The site contains access to free newsletters and RSS feeds to alert
viewers of specific-interest content.)

Medscape
www.medscape.com
((This site offers specialists, primary care physicians, and other health
professionals robust and integrated medical information and educational
tools. The site has the facility to automatically deliver specialty information
that best fits each reader's profile.)

Medline Plus

http://medlineplus.gov
(Site brings together authoritative information from
the National Library of Medicine [NLM], the National Institutes of Health
[NIH], and other government agencies and health-related organizations.
Preformulated searches are included in the site; these allow for easy access
to medical journal articles. The site also has extensive information about
drugs, an illustrated medical encyclopedia, interactive patient tutorials, and
the latest health news.)

Mayo Clinic

Education and Research
www.mayo.edu
(This site explores the world of medical research and education at Mayo Clinic.
It provides information on laboratory and clinical trials, features blogs, and
provides links to publications on a wide range of weight-related topics.)

MedHelp

www.medhelp.org
(This Web site contains over 15 years of accumulated information from
doctors and other patients across hundreds of conditions. In addition, the
site has long-standing partnerships with the top medical institutions such as
the Cleveland Clinic, National Jewish Partners Health, and Mount Sinai.)

ObesityHelp

www.obesityhelp.com
(This site was founded as a peer-support community to help those faced with
life-threatening morbid obesity.

WebMD

www.webmd.com
(This site blends expertise in medicine, journalism, health communication,
and content creation to bring some of the most robust information
possible. MedicineNet.com is a frequent contributor to WebMD and
comprises the Medical Editorial Board. The site also has an independent
medical review board that continuously oversees and reviews the site for
accuracy and timeliness.)

Cancer Organizations

Albert Einstein Cancer Center (AECC)
1300 Morris Park Ave., Bronx, NY 10461
718-430-2000   www.aecom.yu.edu/cancer

American Cancer Society
Atlanta, GA
1-800-227-2345   www.cancer.org

Cancer Care, Inc.
275 Seventh Ave., Fl. 22, New York, NY 10001
800-813-4673   www.cancercare.org

National Cancer Institute (NCI)
Office of Cancer Communications
9000 Rockville Pike, Bldg. 31, Rm. 10A-24, Bethesda, MD 20892
800-422-6237   www.nci.nih.gov

Cardiology Organizations

American College of Cardiology
Heart House, 2400 N. St., N.W., Washington, DC 20037
202-375-6000   www.acc.org

American Heart Association
7272 Greenville Ave., Dallas, TX 75231-4596
214-706-1220   www.americanheart.org

American Stroke Association
7272 Greenville Ave., Dallas, TX 75231
800-478-7653   www.strokeassociation.org

Heart Failure Society of America
Court International, Ste. 240 S, 2550 University Ave. West,
Saint Paul, MN 55114
651-642-1502   www.hfsa.org

National Heart, Lung and Blood Institute
Education Programs Information Center
P.O. Box 30105, Bethesda, MD 20824-0105
301-251-1222   www.nhlbi.nih.gov

Hypertension Network, Inc.
www.bloodpressure.com

Vascular Disease Foundation
1075 S. Yukon, Ste. 320, Lakewood, CO 80226
303-989-0500   www.vdf.org

Diabetes Organizations

American Association of Diabetes Educators (AADE)
200 W. Madison St., Ste. 800, Chicago, IL 60606
800-338-3633   www.diabeteseducator.org

American Diabetic Association
216 W. Jackson Blvd., Chicago, IL 60606-6995
312-899-0040   www.diabetes.org

National Diabetes Education Program
One Diabetes Wy., Bethesda, MD 20814-9692
301-496-3583   www.ndep.nih.gov

Centers for Disease Control and Prevention (CDC)
Division of Diabetes
Translation
4770 Buford Highway N.E., M.S. K-10, Atlanta, GA 30341-3717
770-488-5000   www.cdc.gov/diabetes

Joslin Diabetes Center
One Joslin Place, Boston, MA 02215
617-732-2400   www.joslin.org

Juvenile Diabetes Research Foundation International
120 Wall St., New York, NY 10005-4001
800-533-2873   www.jdrf.org

**National Institute of Diabetes and Digestive and
Kidney Diseases (NIDDK)**
31 Center Dr. MSC-2560, Blvd. 31, Rm. 9A-04, Bethesda, MD 20892-2560
301-496-7422   www.niddk.nih.gov

State of Diabetes Complications in America
888-825-5249   www.stateofdiabetes.com

Dietetic Organizations

American Dietetic Association
120 South Riverside Plaza, Ste. 2000, Chicago, Illinois 60606-6995

Eating Disorders Organizations

American Anorexia/Bulimia Association
165 W, 46th St., Ste. 1108, New York, NY 10036
212-575-6200   www.aabainc.org

Eating Disorders Awareness and Prevention, Inc.
603 Stewart St. Ste. 803, Seattle, WA 98101
206-382-3587   www.edap.org

National Association of Anorexia Nervosa and Associated Disorders
P.O. Box 7, Highland Park, IL 60035
847-381-3438   www.anad.org

National Eating Disorders Association
6655 S. Yale Ave., Tulsa, OK 74136
918-481-4044   www.nationaleatingdisorders.org

Endocrine Organizations

American Association of Clinical Endocrinologists
245 Riverside Ave, Ste. 200, Jacksonville, FL 32202
904-353-7878   www.aace.com

Pediatric Endocrinology Nursing Society (PENS)
PENS National Office, 7794 Grow Dr., Pensacola, FL 32514
1-877-936-7367   www.pens.org

Society for Endocrinology
22 Apex Ct., Woodlands, Bradley Stoke, Bristol BS32 4JT, UK
44-0-1454-642200   www.endocrinology.org

The Endocrine Society
401 Connecticut Ave., Ste. 900 Chevy Chase, MD 20815
301-941-0200   www.endo-society.org

Gynecology & Gastrointestinal Organizations

American Gastroenterological Association
4930 Del Ray Ave., Bethesda, MD 20814
301-654-2055   www.gastro.org

American Gynecological & Obstetrical Society
409 12th St. S.W., Washington, DC 20024
202-863-1647   http://www.agosonline.org

American Society for Gastrointestinal Endoscopy
1520 Kensington Rd., Ste. 202, Oak Brook, IL 60523
866-353-2743   www.asge.org/

Gastroesophageal Reflux Disease (GERD) Organizations

American College of Gastroenterology
P.O. Box 342260, Bethesda, MD 20827-2260
301-263-9000   www.acg.gi.org

American Gastroenterological Association
4930 Del Ray Ave., Bethesda, MD 20814
301-654-2055   www.gastro.org

National Digestive Diseases information Clearinghouse
Two Information Wy., Bethesda, MD 20892–3570
800-891-5389   www.digestive.niddk.nih.gov

Hypertension Organizations

American Society of Hypertension, Inc. (ASH)
148 Madison Ave., Fifth Fl., New York, NY 10016
212-696-9099   www.ash-us.org

International Society of Hypertension (ISH)
ISH Secretariat, Hampton Medical Conferences Ltd., 113-119 High St.
Hampton Hill, Middlesex, TW12 1NJ, U.K.
44-0-20-8979-8300   www.ish-world.com

Pulmonary Hypertension Association (PHA)
801 Roeder Rd., Ste 400, Silver Spring, MD 20910
301-565-3004   www.phassociation.org

Library Journals

Free Medical Journals
www.freemedicaljournals.com

JAMA & ARCHIVES
Subscriber Services Center
American Medical Association
P.O. Box 10946, Chicago, IL 60654
800-262-2350   www.pubs.ama-assn.org

JournalWATCH
860 Winter St., Waltham, MA 02451-1413
781-893-3800   www.jwatch.org

National Agricultural Library
United States Department of Agriculture
Food and Nutrition Information Center
National Agricultural Library
10301 Baltimore Ave., Rm. 105, Beltsville, MD 20705
301-504-5414   www.nal.usda.gov

The Merck Manual: Online Medical Library
www.merck.com/mmpe/index.html

The New England Journal of Medicine
860 Winter St., Waltham, MA 02451-1413
800-843-6356   www.content.nejm.org
United States National Library of Medicine (NLM)
National Institutes of Health
8600 Rockville Pike, Bethesda, MD 20894
301-594-5983   www.nlm.nih.gov

Medication Organizations

RxList
www.rxlist.com/script/main/hp.asp

WebMD
www.webmd.com/drugs/index-drugs.aspx

Nutrition Organizations

American Society for Nutrition
9650 Rockville Pike, Bethesda, MD 20814
301-634-7050   www.nutrition.org

Nutrition.gov
National Agricultural Library
Food and Nutrition Information Center Nutrition.gov Staff,
10301 Baltimore Ave., Beltsville, MD 20705-2351
www.nutrition.gov

Society for Nutrition Education (SNE)
9100 Purdue Rd., Ste. 200, Indianapolis, IN 46268
317-328-4627 www.sne.org

Neurology Organizations

American Neurological Association
5841 Cedar Lake Rd., Ste. 204, Minneapolis, MN 55416
952-545-6284 www.aneuroa.org

Orthopedic Organizations

American Academy of Orthopedic Surgeons (AAOS)
6300 North River Rd., Rosemont, Illinois 60018-4262
847-823-7186 www.aaos.org

American College of Sports Medicine
P.O. Box 1440, Indianapolis, IN 46206-1440
317-637-9200 www.acsm.org

Clinical Orthopedic Society (COS)
2209 Dickens Rd., Richmond, VA 23230-2005
804-565-6366 www.cosociety.org

Obesity Organizations

North American Association for the Study of Obesity (NAASO)
The Obesity Society (AOA)
8630 Fenton St., Ste. 814, Silver Spring, MD 20910
301-563-6526 www.obesity.org

Shape Up America
15009 Native Dancer Rd., North Potomac, MD 20878
www.shapeup.org

The Practical Guide to the Identification, Evaluation and Treatment of Overweight and Obesity in Adults Obesity Research
1090 Amsterdam Ave., Ste. 14K, New York, NY 10025
September 1998 Supplement

Pediatric Organizations

American Academy of Pediatrics
141 Northwest Point Blvd., Elk Grove Village, IL 60007-1098
847-434-4000   www.aap.org

HealthCorps
191 Seventh Ave., #2 N, New York, NY 10011-1818
212-742-2875   www.healthcorps.net

National Childhood Obesity Foundation
N.C.O.F.®
Eleven Hathaway Rd., Ste. 1A, Marblehead, MA 01945
781-639-0048   http://www.ncof.org

Obesity Prevention Foundation
645 N. Arlington Ave., Ste. 525, Reno, NV 89503
775-789-9198   www.obesitypreventionfoundation.org

Red Apple Foundation
P.O. Box 17, West Point, PA 19486
215-699-1726   www.redapplefoundation.org

Plastic Surgery Organizations

National Plastic Surgery Information Center
American Society of Plastic Surgery
444 E. Algonquin Rd., Arlington Heights, IL 60005
800-625-0635

Psychological & Psychiatric Organizations

American Academy of Child & Adolescent Psychiatry
3615 Wisconsin Ave., N.W., Washington, D.C.20016-3007
202-966-2891   www.aacap.org

American Psychiatric Association
1000 Wilson Blvd., Ste. 1825, Arlington, VA 22209
800-357-7924   www.psych.org

American Psychological Association (APA)
750 First St., N.E., Washington, DC 20002-4242
800-374-2721   www.apa.org

Depression and Bipolar Support Alliance (DBSA)
730 N. Franklin St., Ste. 501, Chicago, IL 60610-7224
800-826-3632   www.dbsalliance.org

Mental Health America
2000 N. Beauregard St., 6th Fl., Alexandria, VA 22311
703-684-7722   www.mentalhealthamerica.net

National Alliance on Mental Illness (NAMI)
Colonial Place Three, 2107 Wilson Blvd., Ste. 300, Arlington, VA 22201-3042
703-524-7600   www.nami.org

National Institute of Mental Health
Science Writing, Press and Dissemination Branch
6001 Executive Blvd., Rm. 8184, MSC 9663
Bethesda, MD 20892
301-443-4513   www.nimh.nih.gov

National Mental Health Association
1201 Prince St., Alexandria, VA 22314-2971
800-969-6642   www.nmha.org

Sleep Apnea Organizations

American Sleep Apnea Association (ASAA)
6856 Eastern Ave., N.W., Ste. 203, Washington, DC 20012
202-293-3650   www.sleepapnea.org

National Sleep Foundation
1522 K St., N.W., Ste. 500, Washington, DC 20005
202-347-3472   http://www.sleepfoundation.org

University Organizations
Each of these institutions is a leader in the field of weight loss and
weight management. These organizations' Web sites are useful sources
of information.

DukeHealth.org
Duke Diet Center, 501 Douglas St., Durham, North Carolina 27705
919-688-3079   www.cfl.duke.edu

Penn Medicine: Center for Weight and Eating Disorders
3535 Market St., Ste. 3108, Philadelphia, PA 19104
215-898-2878   www.med.upenn.edu/weight/research

University of Arkansas for Medical Sciences (UAMS)
4301 W. Markham St., Little Rock, AR 72205
501-603-1497   www.weight.uams.edu/

University of Illinois Medical Center
Nutrition and Wellness Center (MC531) 1801 West Taylor St., Rm. 1C
Chicago, Illinois 60612
800-842-1002   www.uillinoismedcenter.org/content.cfm/weight_loss

Washington University Weight Management Program
4570 Children's Pl., First Fl., St. Louis, Missouri 63110
314-286-2080   www.weightmanagement.wustl.edu

Women's Health Organizations

MGH Center for Women's Mental Health
Perinatal and Reproductive Psychiatry Program Simches Research Building
185 Cambridge St., Ste. 2200, Boston, MA 02114
617-724-7792   www.womensmentalhealth.org

National Women's Health Network
1413 K St., N.W., 4th Fl., Washington, DC 20005
202-628-2640   www.womenshealthnetwork.org

National Women's Health Resource Center
157 Broad St., Ste. 106, Red Bank, NJ 07701
800-986-9472   www.healthywomen.org

Sister to Sister: The Women's Heart Health Foundation
4701 Willard Ave., Ste.223, Chevy Chase, MD 20815
301-718-8033   www.sistertosister.org

Timberline Knolls
40 Timberline Dr., Lemont, IL 60439
877-257-9611   www.timberlineknolls.com

Womenshealth.gov
U.S. Department of Health & Human Services
800-994-9662   www.womenshealth.gov

WomenHeart: National Coalition for Women with Heart Disease
818 18th St., N.W., Ste. 930, Washington, DC 20006
202-728-7199   www.womenheart.org

Women's Health Initiative (WHI)
Two Rockledge Ctr., Ste. 10018, Bethesda, MD 20892-7936
301-402-2900   www.nhlbi.nih.gov/whi

Women's Heart Foundation
P.O. Box 7827, West Trenton, NJ 08628
609-771-3778   www.womensheart.org

Women's Place at the University of Virginia
P.O. Box 800566, Charlottesville, VA 22908
434-982-3678   www.healthsystem.virginia.edu/internet/women

About the Author

Kent Sasse, MD, MPH, FACS, is a nationally renowned authority on surgical weight-loss procedures and a leader in the rapidly evolving field of bariatric surgery. The distinguished recipient of several awards, including membership in the prestigious Alpha Omega Alpha Society for top medical graduates in the country, Dr. Sasse is founder and medical director of both the iMetabolic International Metabolic Institute and Western Bariatric Institute, a nationally recognized ASMBS Center of Excellence.

The recipient of a bachelor's degree in biochemistry at the University of California San Diego, where he graduated cum laude, and two master's degrees, including a master's degree in public health stemming from research related to biostatistics and bioethics, from the University of California Berkeley, Dr. Sasse completed residency training in surgery, focusing on gastrointestinal surgery and physiology, at the University of California San Francisco, as well as fellowship training at the Lahey Clinic in Boston, Massachusetts, before establishing his practice in northern Nevada.

Dedicated to the highest levels of scientific research and individualized, state-of-the-art treatment of patients, Dr. Sasse brings a wealth of experience and expertise to the rapidly evolving field of weight-loss surgery. He has written and continues to pursue several IRB-approved research protocols regarding weight loss and weight-loss surgery, and he lectures frequently on topics related to obesity and weight reduction at the University of Nevada School of Medicine. Through his nationally recognized programs, Dr. Sasse and his outstanding faculty provide patients the highest levels of compassionate medicine, scientific evidence, and personalized care in the field of weight reduction.

Dr. Sasse was, until recently, a United States Air Force 9026th Air Reserve Squadron attending surgeon at the Malcolm Grow Medical Center located at Andrews Air Force Base in Maryland. He is the author of numerous books and publications, audio programs, newsletters and a Web site, and he is a featured national speaker in the field of weight loss, bariatric medicine, and weight-loss surgical procedures. He lectures frequently at the University of Nevada School of Medicine on topics related to weight loss and obesity.

Dr. Sasse is the founder of the Obesity Prevention Foundation, a nonprofit foundation dedicated to the prevention of obesity and excessive weight gain in children. Together with Drs. Robert Watson, John Ganser, and Mark Kozar, Dr. Sasse works through the foundation to perform school programs and outreach to parents, teachers, and kids to provide tools to prevent obesity. Visit www.ObesityPrevention.org to learn more.

Please visit www.sasseguide.com for more information on Dr. Sasse and his world-renowned programs and facilities.

Doctor's Orders
101 Medically Proven Tips for Losing Weight
Kent Sasse, MD, MPH, FACS

This simple yet powerful tips resource provides meaningful evidence-based practical and effective tips for initial weight loss and long-term weight maintenance. It touches on key topics that help remind readers to initiate and ingrain long-term healthy behaviors. It points out small meaningful steps that each person can all take on the road to a healthier weight. Readers can take advantage of Dr. Sasse's insight and reading of the scientific literature to make the weight loss journey a success.

Outpatient Weight-Loss Surgery
Safe and Successful Weight Loss with Modern Bariatric Surgery
Kent Sasse, MD, MPH, FACS

Written in clear, direct, easy-to-follow language and containing real-life personal stories, educational illustrations, and a comprehensive resource section, this book is an invaluable resource for the medical community and anyone considering a bariatric surgical procedure today.

Ditch Your Diet in 30 Days
90 Easy, Healthy Meal and Snack Recipes for Effective Weight Loss
Chef Dave Fouts and Vicki Bovee, MS, RD

This cookbook provides a systematic meal plan for 30 days. It provides recipes for five meals per day that allow the reader to maintain a 1,200-calorie-per-day intake routine. From shopping lists to complete nutritional panels, this cookbook provides everything needed to bring variety, nutritional balance, and delicious meals not only to those who have had bariatric surgery, but also to anyone else who is seeking delicious meal ideas that help maintain proper nutritional balance.

Shakin' It Up
Chef Dave Fouts with Nutritional Consultation by Vicki Bovee, MS, RD

This recipe book delivers wonderful and creative shake recipes from a trained chef who has undergone bariatric surgery himself and who understands the need for diversity and flavor during this very important phases before and after surgery. In addition, this book is valuable to anyone making meal replacements a normal part of a weight-loss or weight-maintenance routine.

Smooth Foods
Chef Dave Fouts with Nutritional Consultation by Vicki Bovee, MS, RD

This recipe book focuses on the second eating phase after weight loss surgery, when smooth, easy-to-digest foods are the order of the day. Chef Dave Fouts provides recipes that are geared toward providing variety and sound nutrition while fulfilling protein, vitamin, and texture needs of anyone who has undergone weight-loss surgery.

E-BOOKS

Adolescents and Weight-Loss Surgery: The Benefits and Risks

Seniors and Weight-Loss Surgery: The Benefits and Risks

Which Weight-Loss Procedure Is Right For Me?: The Latest Data on Bariatric Surgery Helps You Decide

After Weight Loss Surgery: The Keys to Weight-Loss Success After Bariatric Surgery

Index